Contents

Preface   vii

Onset of Stuttering: The Case of the Missing Block
William H. Perkins, PhD   1

Continuity, Fragmentation, and Tension:
   Hypotheses Applied to Evaluation and Intervention with
   Preschool Disfluent Children
David Prins, PhD   21

Evaluation as a Basis for Intervention
Glyndon Riley, PhD
Jeanna Riley, MA, CCC   43

Current Behavioral Treatments for Children
Janis M. Costello, PhD   60

Spontaneous Remission of Stuttering:
   When Will the Emperor Realize He Has No Clothes On?
Roger J. Ingham, PhD 113

Issues and Perspectives
David Prins, PhD
Roger J. Ingham, PhD 141

Index 147

Preface

The first five chapters are based on papers presented at a regional conference hosted in Seattle by the Department of Speech and Hearing Sciences, University of Washington, March 4-6, 1982.

The conference was intended, as is the text, for would-be and practicing clinicians and educators who are concerned about the problem of stuttering, its origins in young children, and the bases and procedures for intervention.

Four major topics are considered:

The nature of disfluent speech and of the disfluencies that characterize stuttering;

The evaluation of speech and other factors that form the bases for clinical intervention;

Therapy techniques for working directly on fluency enhancement with young children;

Recovery and outcome.

In the chapters that follow, these topics are dealt with more or less in the order presented, and by a group of authors with diverse backgrounds and sometimes conflicting points of view.

The paper by William Perkins served to keynote the conference. Through an imaginative process of deductive inference, it speculates on the fundamental nature of the fluency failures that lead to stuttering. The questions it raises ultimately concern the origin and definition of stuttering and factors that could be essential to its evaluation, prevention, and treatment. It is through these latter factors that this chapter is linked to others in this volume.

David Prins' chapter deals with the linguistic origins of disfluency, factors that may be associated with the development of disfluency into the symptoms that characterize stuttering, and applications of this information to clinical intervention decisions with preschool children.

In their chapter, Glyndon and Jeanna Riley review a multiple component model for evaluation and intervention. They emphasize the assessment of different factors that can contribute to stuttering and the differential programming of treatment based on these factors. The chapter highlights the need to view stuttering as a disorder with multiple etiologic and maintaining factors.

Janis Costello, in her chapter, deals primarily with the procedures and techniques of behavior modification to shape and maintain speech fluency. Specific programming strategies are summarized that deal with the sequence of activities and the use of reinforcement.

In his chapter on spontaneous remission of stuttering, Roger Ingham reviews critically the design and findings of studies of the so-called self-recovery of stuttering. His conclusions shed quite a different light on the literature which generally has been taken to mean that "untreated" stuttering is very apt to resolve itself.

The conference format was designed to permit maximum interaction between the presenters and conferees. Following each paper, the audience was divided into four seminar groups that met for about one hour to discuss the paper and raise questions. The audience then reassembled, and the group leaders were given an opportunity to address their groups' questions to the presenter. Selected questions and answers from these sessions are included following each of the individually authored chapters.

The last chapter, completed following the conference, serves to highlight and put into perspective the major issues and positions taken.

ACKNOWLEDGMENT

The papers in this text were given at a conference sponsored by the Department of Speech and Hearing Sciences, University of Washington, and by funds from the Office of Education, Bureau of Education for the Handicapped. Many faculty and staff members of the Department participated to help make the conference possible. Special contributions were made by:

Dr. Fred D. Minifie, Chairman, Department of Speech and Hearing Sciences

Dr. F. Ann Cerf, moderator of post-presentation discussions

Mr. Kenneth Griesser, audio-visual media coordinator

Ms. Karen Iwamoto and Mr. Howard Goldsmith, tape transcribers for discussion sessions

TREATMENT OF STUTTERING IN EARLY CHILDHOOD

methods and issues

David Prins
Roger J. Ingham

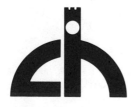

College-Hill Press • San Diego, California

College-Hill Press, Inc.
4284 41st Street
San Diego, California 92105

Library of Congress Cataloging in Publication Data
Main entry under title:

Treatment of stuttering in early childhood.

  The first five chapters are based on papers presented at a regional conference hosted in Seattle by the Department of Speech and Hearing Sciences, University of Washington, March 4-6, 1982.
  Includes bibliographical references and index.
  1. Stuttering in children—Congresses. I. Prins, David   II. Ingham, Roger J.
[DNLM: 1. Stuttering—In infancy and childhood—Congresses.   2. Stuttering—Therapy—Congresses.
WM 475 T784 1982]
RJ496.S8T73 1982   618.92'8554   82-17914
ISBN 0-933014-79-1

Printed in the United States of America

1

Onset of Stuttering: The Case of the Missing Block

William H. Perkins
University of Southern California

For those of you familiar with Nero Wolfe mystery novels, I would like to attribute current explanations of stuttering to the work of Archie, Nero's right hand man. Archie is an astute observer, but invariably misses the critical bit of evidence. With apologies to Rex Stout, Nero's creator, and to you (especially if you've never heard of Nero), may we look at the onset of stuttering as Nero might see it. I have a strong suspicion that the way we have assembled our blocks of evidence would not make sense to him. If I am right, then we probably have before us most of the parts we need to build a solution to the mystery of why stuttering develops as it does. The question for us is which of these blocks that we Archies have been looking at, and missing, for years is the one that Nero would spot as the key to our answer. So let us pretend that a Society To Understand Fluency Findings has been recently formed and has asked Nero for guidance. And let us pretend further that Nero has sent Archie out to gather facts.

The "crime" that Nero has been commissioned to solve is why, out of all of the children who ever stutter, will about three-fourths recover, and will about one-fourth struggle with the problem for much of their lives? What do we know about this "crime?"

STUTTERING DEFINED

First, we know reasonably well what people do when they are heard to stutter. Wendell Johnson cast stuttering in the broader framework of disfluency for which he devised an eight-category classification system. Of course, normal speakers use some of these categories, such as phrase repetitions, revisions, incomplete phrases, and interjections, as much as do stutterers, so these types of disfluency do not appear to tell us much about stuttering. On the other hand, part-word repetitions and prolonged sounds are far more likely to be found in stuttered than in normal speech; so much so, in fact, that many of us have taken the disfluent syllable as our operational definition of stuttering. Others of us, however, are not too satisfied with this definition for several reasons. For one thing, it is too fine a net with which to catch only stuttering; after all, normal speakers repeat syllables, too. For another, this definition is too exclusive; only sounds, not syllables, can be prolonged either audibly or silently (as in a hesitation). Some of us, therefore, have opted for the disfluent sound as our operational definition of stuttering, and some, such as Wingate (1969), have refined it to the level of a phonetic transition disfluency. Drawing on Wingate, Andrews' (1981) conclusion about a consensus definition of stuttering is that repetitions and prolongations of sounds or syllables are necessary and sufficent for a diagnosis of stuttering. Unfortunately, these definitions, too, have their problems, not the least of which is that normal speakers also hesitate, repeat, and prolong sounds. The troublesome fact is that, when it comes to defining stuttering, stutterers do not do anything observable which normal speakers do not also do. They may not do some of them as frequently as do stutterers, but they still do them.

Another feature of our "crime" is that we know who the witnesses have been. They have been the subjects in our clinical and laboratory attempts to define stuttering. Paraphrasing Bloodstein (1981), stuttering is defined as whatever is perceived as stuttering by reliable observers whose judgments agree. Ironically, this tends to exclude stutterers from judgments of their own stuttering. The reasoning is that because they respond to subjective perceptions of their own stuttering to which other listeners are not privy, judgments of their own speech are less likely to agree with those of reliable observers. On the other hand, their judgments of the stuttering of others may be just as reliable as those of any other objective judge. Thus, we Archies have insisted on reliable witnesses. We are not about to become soft-headed and succumb to unverified observations.

If listeners can make reliable judgments of stuttering, then there must be some characteristics of disfluency on which they base these judgments. Indeed, there are. Disfluencies that last more than a second, occur on more than three percent of syllables spoken, involve two or more sound or syllable repetitions, and show signs of struggle are likely to be judged as stuttering. There is a catch to these "reliable" judgments, however. High agreement is found only when you ask listeners to count the total number of stutterings they hear. If you ask them to compare specific instances of stuttering, even if they compare their own judgments from one day to the next, they will be lucky to be in agreement half of the time. The sum of the matter is that even though we seem to think that we can detect how much stuttering occurs, the distinction between normal and stuttered disfluencies is remarkably muddy (Curlee, 1981).

Do we know any more about who is a stutterer than we do about what stuttering is? The answer is debatable. Ironically, calling a person a stutterer changes our judgments of his stuttering. Repetitions, pauses, circumlocutions that would otherwise pass as normal disfluencies are likely to be heard as integral parts of stuttering if the speaker is thought to be a stutterer who is trying to avoid stuttering. The problem of deciding who is a stutterer has another complication to it as well. Some people who complain bitterly about being stutterers are rarely, if ever, heard to stutter. What do we make of them? How can they be stutterers if they don't stutter? And yet, they are convinced that stuttering is a paralyzing problem for them. Despite these reservations, we seem to agree reasonably well on who we think is a stutterer, except with young children for whom that judgment is shaky.

DEVELOPMENT OF STUTTERING

Beyond our definitions of stuttering and stutterer, what do we know about how stuttering develops? Bloodstein (1960) has observed that it goes through four phases. In most cases, it begins between ages two and six, which suggests that it begins after the child has mastered enough language skills to speak his ideas rapidly enough to keep up with a conversation. I will only highlight salient features of each phase.

In Phase One, the interruptions tend to be repetitions; they tend to be episodic for periods of weeks or months, interspersed with long interludes of normal fluency; they tend to occur when excited or under communicative pressure; and children seem unaware of most of their interruptions, except when stuck in an effort to communicate — then they react with acute frustration, but they do not appear to think of themselves as stutterers. Phase Two corresponds roughly to elementary school age. In this phase, they tend to regard themselves as stutterers, but they still have little concern for their interruptions; they stutter chiefly when excited or talking fast; and the stuttering has become chronic. Phase Three is most common in late childhood and early adolescence. The person still speaks freely with little avoidance, fear, or embarrassment despite severe blockages to which he may react with irritation. Finally, with Phase Four comes the full-blown clinical problem of stuttering, which may be seen as early as ten years of age, but typically occurs later. With it come shame, anxiety, fear and avoidance of stuttering and speaking, and acute consciousness of how listeners react.

CHARACTERISTICS OF STUTTERERS

What can we say with any certainty about the stutterer? Certainly he has been probed and punctured in every conceivable corner of his soma and psyche for any difference to which we could point as the cause of his stuttering. As matters stand, the best we can say is that whatever the cause turns out to be, it will have something to do with being inherited and with factors favoring males. The greater prevalence of stuttering among males than females consistently turns up at a ratio of 3:1 to 4:1. As for inheritance, both genetic and environmental factors seem to be involved. Kidd's (1980) extensive genetic studies lead to this conclusion, as does Howie's (1981) study of identical and fraternal same-sex twins. If one of a pair of monozygotic twins stutters, there is 77 percent probability that the other twin will stutter, even if he has been raised separately. With dizygotic same-sex twins, the risk drops to 32 percent. Thus, it is possible for genetic transmission of some biological characteristic to account in some cases for most, but probably not all, of stuttering. Were the cause wholly transmitted genetically, then if stuttering were found in one identical twin, it would always be found in the other, but in one-fourth of the cases, this does not occur. Whether stuttering can result from environmental factors in the absence of genetic inheritance is not as clear.

Much has been made in recent years about differences between stutterers and nonstutterers in laryngeal functioning, to say nothing about differences in brain functioning and auditory functioning. Not too much can be made of these differences for several reasons. First, many stutterers do not show these differences, and many of the differences are so small as to be found only with sophisticated statistical manipulations. To talk about the cause of stuttering in any given individual on the basis of small group differences is hazardous. Second, most of these differences have been turned up in adults whose experience of stuttering may have had as much to do with causing them as of being caused by them. Which leads to another reservation. To say that any of these differences cause stuttering is equivalent to saying that winter occurs because trees shed brown leaves in the fall. The observed differences between stutterers and nonstutterers only suggest possible causes. Until stuttering is observed to vary with manipulation of these differences, attributing cause to them is premature speculation.

STUTTERING AS A RESPONSE

A multitude of conditions have been associated with reduction of stuttering. A few will invariably eliminate it immediately, such as lipped speech, prolonged articulation, and probably rhythmic speech, singing, and shadow reading. Some will usually reduce it immediately, such as whispering, masking, speaking alone, adaptation readings, and response-contingent punishment. But the majority, such as linguistic factors, only reduce it for some stutterers part of the time and not very much. Lest we get too excited about finding an easy answer among these conditions, let me caution you that they have the same effects on the disfluencies of normal speakers as they have on the disfluencies of stutterers.

Other conditions have been associated with increases in stuttering, such as communicative responsibility and time pressure, audience size, concern about social approval, general anxiety about speech, and expectation of stuttering on certain sounds and words in certain situations. Some of these conditions may play a role in onset of stuttering, but what that role may be is still a matter for conjecture; it has not been clearly demonstrated. One of these conditions has at least been delimited, however. The ability to predict when stuttering will occur is a characteristic of chronic stutterers and does not appear until later stages of development of stuttering, so it can not very well be a factor in initial phases of onset.

THEORIES OF STUTTERING

You Nero and Archie fans know, of course, that Archie does all of the legwork while Nero putters with his orchids and tells him where to look. Nero only wants the main facts, the big picture, to begin his ruminations, so the foregoing report, let us say, is what Archie might have presented to him My guess is that Nero's reply would be, "My, those people seem to know a lot about stuttering, but I gather that they still don't know what causes it. Remarkable. Surely, they have tried to assemble these facts into answers." To which Archie replies, "Have they ever! The main theory for years, which still has a lot of support, stems from Wendell Johnson's argument that stuttering begins in the ear of the listener, usually a parent, who thinks that the normal disfluencies of the child are instances of stuttering. As the parent becomes concerned, so does the child, who, by hesitating to hesitate, learns to struggle with disfluencies in an attempt to be fluent. Thus, Johnson thought that the abnormalities of stuttered speech are what the normal speaking child learns to do in order to avoid doing what his parents think is stuttering.

Nero then asks a question that launches the following conversation.

Nero: Are children who stutter insecure?

Archie: I'm sure some are, but as a group, they seem to be as secure as normal-speaking children.

Nero: What about parents? Are they exceptionally protective or punishing?

Archie: The evidence is mixed, but I couldn't find a clear difference.

Nero: Curious, why would a child react to punishment of his disfluency with increased disfluency when the consequence of punishment is a reduction of contingent behavior? Another problem with this theory is that it doesn't explain why a few normally disfluent children who are no more insecure than most, and whose parents are not exceptionally different, will become severe chronic stutterers. If they or their parents are no different, why would only they learn to stutter?

Archie: Well, those who followed Johnson have had difficulty with his theory, too. Bloodstein's (1981) version is a proposal that when the normal tensions and fragmentations of speech of young children are monstrified by communicative pressure, they become stutterers. Others think that stuttering is an operant response that develops and is preserved by contingent reinforcement.

Nero: Perhaps, but neither explanation accounts for why only a few normal children will become stutterers, unless you can show me evidence that they have been under prolonged, unusually powerful communicative stress and have had resultant disfluencies strongly reinforced.

Archie: So far as I found, normal-speaking children have to cope with about the same pressures and reinforcements.

Nero: Hmmmm.

Archie: Another possibility is Brutten's (1967) idea that the core repetitions and prolongations are disruptions of fluency caused by nonspecific stress and anxiety.

Nero: Well, are young stutterers more anxious than non-stutterers? Will stress on normal-speaking children produce abnormal sound or syllable disfluency? And what about adult stutterers; do they only have trouble when anxious or under stress?

Archie: Not so far as I could find.

Nero: I am not persuaded that learning alone can account for stuttering. I presume that someone must think that incipient stutterers have inherited a biological proclivity to stutter.

Archie: Many do, but they have had little success finding what that proclivity might be. The fact that genetic transmission can play a major role is the most persuasive reason for suspecting an organic basis. Some are convinced that laryngeal coordinations are pivotally involved, mainly because stuttering varies consistently with manipulations of the complexity of laryngeal coordinations, but not with vocal tract coordinations. The problem has to be in the motor control system. If it were in the larynx itself, then a laryngectomy should invariably eliminate stuttering, which it usually does, but not always. Also, any biological explanation must account for why most stutterers are fluent more of the time than they stutter.

Nero: Obviously, they are considering the brain, but that's a vast territory.

Archie: It sure is, but most of the evidence indicates that motor speech planning takes longer for stutterers than non-stutterers. Mainly, the scientists are looking for answers in cortical motor planning operations, brain stem reflex coordination mechanisms, and auditory feedback systems. Certainly delayed auditory feedback is known to disrupt fluency, but stutterers say that the disruptions are different from stuttering. Also, all of the hypotheses proposed apply as much to the disfluencies of normal speakers as to those of stutterers. I just don't see how any of these answers could explain why only a few children are ever thought to stutter, and of these, why only a fourth will carry chronic stuttering into adulthood. And what about severe stutterers who recover, sometimes almost overnight? Or better yet, what about the adult who decides he's tired of stuttering and quits — literally? If their stuttering were a consequence of some constitutional defect, how could they become normally fluent if the defect were not corrected?

Nero: Archie, you wear me out.

With that remark, Nero picked up his potting tool and returned to his orchids. The next Archie heard from him was an urgent summons to Nero's study.

Nero: Archie, I think the answer is at hand. I want you to do some detecting. First, check any definition of stuttering you can find that would tell me what a stutterer does that he himself thinks is stuttering. Then find out if stutterers can volitionally do what they think is stuttering. Also, I need to know why stutterers who never stutter think that they are stutterers. Finally, you will need to search the literature for any longitudinal studies of very young stutterers who became chronic stutterers.

Archie: I suppose you want this by day before yesterday.

Nero: No, no, this afternoon will be fine. Oh, I almost forgot; borrow a DAF unit (I hate acronyms) and see for yourself what it does to speech. Try it on a couple of dozen children and adults. Include some who stutter severely, some who are mild, and some who've

never stuttered. And find out as much about auditory feedback
as you can.
A week later, Archie reports back.
Nero: You certainly took long enough. Don't apologize. Just give me the
facts.

Archie spent the next two hours reporting his observations and findings,
interrupted here and there by Nero's probes for clarification. Then came
this order.

Nero: Archie, dispatch an invitation to the Society To Understand
Fluency Findings. I detest their acronym, STUFF, but they have
employed us to make sense of their findings, so we will permit
them to choose the time for our report — but I will choose the
place.

All members of STUFF were invited: speech pathologists, psycholo-
gists, neurologists, speech scientists, all with a vested interest in understanding the nature and onset of stuttering.

What follows was Nero's report.

Madam Chairman, Ladies and Gentlemen, You have commissioned
me to find a clue to the onset of stuttering. I am only a detective. I am not
equipped, nor inclined, to engage in experimental research. The only com-
missions I accept are ones I can solve by thinking.
The first thing I will tell you is that I admire your industriousness. I
marvel at the energy you expend investigating even the faintest lead with
research methods that are sometimes extraordinarily sophisticated. I
wonder, though, why you exert yourselves so mightily without thinking
through what your projects could possibly mean.
To sort through your truckloads of facts in search of meaningful clues
about why stuttering develops as it does taxed my endurance. The only
way I could proceed was to determine what answers were excluded. If the
problem were entirely organic, I reasoned, then genetic transmission
would account for it wholly in the majority of cases, and with virtually no
exceptions in identical twins. It does not. If entirely learned, no credible
explanation seems possible that would explain the probability of stuttering
in families of stutterers: 77 percent in identical twins, 32 percent in same-
sex fraternal twins, and 18 percent in same-sex siblings. I therefore concluded that I was looking for an inheritable mechanism of stuttering which
could be triggered by noninherited conditions.
Having no idea what this mechanism might be, nor what it was supposed to do, I searched Archie's report for a clue. Six points leaped forth.

Point One: If you are going to find a biological mechanism to account for stuttering, then I would think you would begin your search with a description of the performance characteristics that the mechanism is supposed to control. Rarely has this happened. Most have started with some known physiological mechanism and have then tried to superimpose it onto stuttering as a possible explanation. I concluded that whatever is known of the mechanism of stuttering is far too speculative for me to use as a starting point, so I then began looking for what it is about stuttering that I am trying to explain. The remaining points then emerged.

Point Two: The types and forms of disfluency that are called stuttering are not observably different from disfluencies of normal speakers. They may occur more frequently and last longer, but even that is not necessarily true.

Point Three: The only thing that seems to categorically separate confirmed stutterers who consider themselves to be stutterers from normal speakers is their apprehensive reaction to stuttering, and this only appears in the final stage of development. The child just beginning to stutter may struggle when stuck, but his struggles seem to be from frustration, not fear.

Point Four: The vast majority of children who are thought to stutter, about 75 percent, will recover before adulthood.

Point Five: The definitions of stuttering that have gained acceptance have all permitted reliable observation of observable behavior.

Point Six: The consensus is that sound or syllable repetitions and prolongations (audible or silent) are necessary and sufficient to define stuttering.

What appeared from these last five points was a glimmering of what I was seeking. It was from these points that I sent Archie on some errands. What he found, coupled with what I already knew from his earlier report, has led me to several conclusions. Probably none of them will win me much popularity with you members of STUFF. This is of no concern; you have paid me only for guidance, not popularity.

My first conclusion is that you prefer a hopeless definition of stuttering. With your consensus definition, you will never separate stutterers from nonstutterers, nor stuttering from normal disfluency. Moreover, your definition is neither necessary nor sufficient. It certainly is not sufficient when the behavior it identifies — repetitions and prolongations — are characteristic of normal disfluency. As for being necessary, it does not define the covert stutterer who develops a vocabulary of synonyms and skill at circumlocution that permits avoidance of stuttering. Archie found several of these men. One in particular was so successful in hiding his stuttering that his wife did not know of it for fifteen years. Yet he and the others like him live in dread of detection. If they do not qualify as stutterers by their apprehension of stuttering, who does?

My second conclusion will be particularly distasteful because it will put your sacred cow, reliability, in jeopardy. I arrived at this conclusion — I will tell you about it momentarily — by asking myself two questions: first, why are stutterers who never stutter convinced that they are constantly at risk of stuttering? And, second, what could possibly happen to a child that could make him so anxious about stuttering that he becomes fearful and ashamed of speaking? If all he does is hesitate, repeat, and prolong sounds, even if he does it more than normally disfluent children, it would likely require monstrous punishment to make all but the most insecure child struggle to avoid those normal disfluencies. It is not an impossible explanation, but it does strain credulity. No, the answer must be simpler, as indeed it appears to be. My second conclusion is that what makes stutterers and stuttering different is the condition of being involuntarily blocked. Unfortunately, for the sake of reliability and verification, this may not be a condition that anyone can detect other than the person who stutters.

This conclusion is pivotal, so permit me some elaboration. Archie's reports from covert stutterers put me onto this track. They told him that if they were not constantly vigilant, they would become hopelessly stuck, which would be acutely embarrassing. They said they did not let their guard down often, but when they did the result was mortifying. This seemed to be a reaction that, if found in beginning stutterers and chronic stutterers, might hold the key that would unlock this puzzle.

I did not have to look far to find confirmation, in fact, the International Classification of Diseases includes this missing block (I use the term literally and figuratively) in its definition: stuttering is a disorder in which the speaker knows what he wishes to say but cannot, for the moment, say it because of *involuntary* repetitions, prolongations, or cessations of sound. Wingate's (1964) standard definition is similar: stuttering "is characterized by involuntary, audible or silent, repetitions or prolongations in the utterance of short speech elements." Ironically, the necessary and sufficient part of these definitions (the involuntary part) seems to be the part that has been omitted from the currently accepted consensus definition.

Next, I considered how stutterers described their own stuttering to Archie. The common theme, exemplified by the frequent comment, "My tongue sticks to the roof of my mouth," is frustration, tension, and apprehension at being literally unable to make the speech organs move through the articulatory positions of the word on which they are stuck. Equally noteworthy were their evaluations of their attempts to imitate their own stuttering. Everyone could distinguish "real" from faked stuttering. When it is real, it is tense and involuntary. Among the more frequent comments were, "It's like I can't control my speech," and "I could stop the fakes when I want to, but not the real ones." Here, then, is something adult stutterers do that is understandably frightening to them.

The critical question remained, though, whether this adult reaction developed as a consequence of apprehension about childhood disfluencies that are essentially normal, or as a cause of fear and struggle. At least part of the answer was in Archie's original report of Bloodstein's studies. Even in the earliest phases of stuttering, severe disruptions are mixed among the predominant repetitions. They are frustrating enough that typical reactions include refusing to speak, complaining of being unable to talk, and crying. As stuttering develops, these irritations with blockage increase until they apparently culminate in the anxiety and shame of clinical stuttering.

So far, so good, although I will soon come to a caveat that you must heed. At least I now have a picture of what the stutterer does that he reacts to so strongly — he loses control and becomes stuck. The question we have now reached is whether he involuntarily blocks because he tenses and struggles to speak. If he does, we would expect his blockages to become progressively more severe as his stuttering develops. This does not seem to happen. His frustration is acute from the beginning, but only as a reaction to stoppages, not to easy repetitions; he appears to struggle tensely in an attempt to cope with being involuntarily blocked. What seems to increase in severity as stuttering develops is not the condition of being stuck in the block, but the frequency of its occurrence and the forcefulness of the struggles to become unstuck.

I began my service to you by narrowing my search. I was reasonably confident that I was looking for an inheritable mechanism of stuttering that could be triggered by noninherited conditions. Now my search was narrowed further, I was no longer looking for a mechanism that would account for any sound or syllable repetition, prolongation, or hesitation. Such a mechanism would account for normal disfluency or stuttering, but it would not separate one from the other. Clearly, stutterers exhibit both types of disfluency. But it is only the involuntary type, not the normal disfluencies, with which they apparently struggle. No, what I was looking for now was evidence of a mechanism that would account for involuntary blockage, and a trigger that could vary from one condition to another.

I looked first for signs that an inheritable mechanism might exist. Mindful of all the recent hubbub about the larynx, I thought that to be a sensible place to start. Aside from some science-fiction publicity announcements that stutterers can find relief from laryngeal spasms if they are willing to live atop the Empire State Building, an abundance of descriptive studies have suggested that laryngeal reaction times are slower in stutterers than nonstutterers. But these differences are small, many stutterers do not exhibit them, and they have not been shown experimentally to vary with stuttering, so I could assign little confidence to them. What did implicate the larynx as possibly being involved in the mechanism of stuttering was an invariant increase in stuttering of 90 percent when laryngeal management of the air stream is changed from lipped speech with no air flow to whispered speech with voiceless air flow. Then, by changing whispering to voiced-voiceless air flow of normal speech, stuttering increases almost 60 percent. What caught my attention most was that no stutterer was found — no matter how severe — out of more than a hundred tested, who had any feeling of stuttering during lipped speech. Many had gross distortions of tongue, lips, and jaw during stuttering spasms, but all of these disappeared immediately during lipped speech.

Was there something about the larynx itself that would explain why it seems to be strongly connected to stuttering? If so, no stutterer who has been laryngectomized should ever stutter again, but this possibility was excluded by the fact that a few laryngectomized stutterers still stutter. It was Archie who gave me an intriguing lead. In his report on auditory feedback, he found a study by Stromsta that links sound blockage to auditory control of the larynx. In 1959, Stromsta elaborated on the work of a French team of investigators led by Vannier who had a technique by which they could block phonation. They did this by delaying normal auditory feedback with a shift of the phase of the fundamental frequency. What Stromsta did was to combine phase shifts with distortion of feedback of sustained vowels. When he only distorted the feedback, intermittent phonatory blockage occurred along with extreme pitch variations and rough voice quality. When he manipulated the phase angle of the fundamental frequency of the distorted vowel, he could produce sustained blockage with particular phase angles. When those angles were shifted, intermittent blockage would recur, only to become sustained again when the original angle was reinstated. This phase angle had to be re-established with each breath, however, because it shifted from one breath to the next. In other words, here were experimental conditions in which normal speakers could be made to block as stutterers do, but on only one vowel at a time, and mainly using a falsetto voice.

In 1972, Stromsta followed this up with an investigation of differences in interaural feedback delay between stutterers and nonstutterers. Although some subjects in these two groups overlapped a bit, they showed remarkably consistent and sizable differences. His experiment did not allow him to connect these differences with stuttering, so I will not yet take the liberty of drawing inferences he did not permit himself to make.

Most of these studies implicating involvement of the larynx in stuttering were done on adults. I wondered, now, if I could find similar evidence of laryngeal involvement in early onset of stuttering. What I found not only linked the larynx to speech blockage in young stutterers, it linked it to the development of chronic stuttering. Again, I am indebted to Dr. Stromsta for providing this evidence. In 1965, he reported on 38 children whose parents thought they stuttered. He made spectrograms of their speech. Of these 38 spectrograms, 27 showed abrupt phonatory stoppages and lacked second formant transitions in connection with prolongations and repetitive blocks. Ten years later, he inquired about these 38 children with a questionnaire. Of the 27 with abnormal spectrograms, 24 were still stuttering. Of the 11 who did not show phonatory stoppages, 10 were now considered to be normal speakers.

Little did I realize how close to home this investigation would lead. I asked Archie to borrow a DAF unit and experiment on its effects. He used it with half a dozen children and more than a dozen adults who had their stuttering under control, but still stuttered when they relaxed those controls. No amount of auditory delay resulted in stuttering with a single one of them. To be sure, they were affected by DAF. Loudness increased, their rates slowed, they became disfluent, but none of these effects resembled stuttering. Only two speakers could be found out of several dozen tested whose reaction to DAF sounded like stuttering. Neither of them has ever stuttered, and one of them is Archie.

I have asked him to demonstrate for you. I have also asked him to fake his DAF-induced disfluencies every now and then so that you may compare what he does volitionally with what he does involuntarily. Would you also note that he can change the topography of his "stuttering" from repetitions to hard blocks to repetitions by changing the pressure to communicate. Finally, please take special note that no blockage occurs if his speech is slow and relaxed. Moreover, any block that does occur can be terminated by slowing his articulatory rate. Archie, will you now speak to us?

Archie: Mr. Wolfe, Ladies and Gentlemen, I am speaking to you now with no auditory delay. I will attempt to maintain this articulatory rate and introduce 50 msec. of au----ditory d-d-d-delay. Th----e effect you n-n-now observe is inv----oluntary. I----I----I have exp-p-perimented with th-th-this d-d-d-device for m-months now and I am st-st-still com-pl-pletely unable to sp-sp-speak at this r-r-rate w-w-without being bl-blocked. Most people can push through it, b----b----but the har-har-harder I t try the m-m-m----ore I inv----vo----luntarily d----d----do what you are ob---s----serving r-r-right now. On the other hand, if I back off on communicative pressure and slow the articulatory movements, the blockage ceases immediately and I feel no effects of DAF or any sense of stickiness in my speech, even though the delay is still set at 50 msec. If I increase the delay to 100 msec. as I just have, then to 150, which is where it is now, and finally to 200, the main effect is to slow the articulatory rate I must use to remain free of blockage. If I exceed the disruption rate limit, I w----w----will be bl-bl----blocked, but no m-m-more severely with one am-m-m-mount of de-de-delay than an-nother. Now I will turn off the delay and simulate the blockages I have been having which I imagine w-w-will n-n-not b-be discernibly d----d----d---different to you, nor to me for th-th-that matter, with one n-n-notable d-d-differ-ence--- I can stop them whenever I wish without slowing down. Is this sufficient, Mr. Wolfe?

Nero: Thank you Archie. Let me be sure I understand what you just did. You turned off the delay you could not beat and faked the remaining blocks, which you were able to stop at any instant and return immediately to rapid speech. Is it not apparent that if the essence of stuttering is involuntary blockage, then the only one privileged to know whether a disfluency is stuttered or not is the stutterer? I think it obvious, Archie, that you could become one of the world's worst stutterers if, with your rapid speech rate, you had to speak continuously under conditions of auditory delay. You have apparently inherited the mechanism for stuttering, but for you, the trigger condition never occurred until I sent you on this DAF assignment. Equally obviously, 50 to 200 msec. of auditory delay does not serve as the trigger for all stutterers, and possibly for none, even though it conceivably could in those stutterers who block on virtually every syllable.

With your demonstration, Archie, you have brought me to the most indeterminant part of my speech. All of the evidence I have seen implicates the laryngeal control system as the inherited mechanism responsible for speech blockage. In all probability, discoordinated movements of the vocal tract articulatory apparatus can also produce repetitions, prolongations, and hesitations, but I find no evidence that these disfluencies involve involuntary blockage. What I do not know with any certainty is the aspect of control that is implicated. Stromsta could block phonation by tinkering with fundamental frequency control, but he had to distort the vowel /u/ and produce it in falsetto to produce blockage. Whether the same results could be obtained with connected speech is not known. For that matter, some other aspect of laryngeal control may be responsible for stuttering blocks. As matters stand, though, I would place my bet on fundamental frequency control and play that hand as far as it could profitably be taken.

Next, I would look for trigger conditions that would account for severe episodes of blocking at the onset of stuttering followed by periods of fluency, and that would account for all of its varying characteristics as it develops into a chronic clinical problem, and that would account for the recovery of severe stutterers into reasonably normal speakers. At least three conditions are apparent candidates. They are probably not mutually exclusive. I warned you when I accepted your commission that I am not equipped to perform laboratory experimentation, so I can not tell you whether these conditions operate independently or interact with each other.

Nor can I be certain, without experimentation, that these are the conditions you seek. I can tell you, however, that were I so inclined, I would begin by investigating interactions between phase angle feedback of fundamental frequency with articulatory rate and with communicative pressure.

Judging from Stromsta's success with blocking phonation in normal speakers, everyone may have inherited a blockage mechanism. If this is the case, then why are these mechanisms more readily triggered in children who become stutterers than in normal-speaking children? The answer may lie in the difference in interaural disparity between stutterers and nonstutterers. In Stromsta's study of 50 male adults, half who stuttered and half who didn't, he found that the normal feedback delay in nonstutterers was 0.3 msec., but in stutterers was over 0.6 msec. at 150 Hz. At higher frequencies, the differences were still highly significant, but considerably smaller.

If you wish to see why this result is deliciously tempting, recall that when Stromsta distorted higher frequencies, phonation was blocked intermittently, but at fundamental frequencies in the neighborhood of 150 Hz, sustained blockage occurred. If that coincidence isn't tempting enough, then add the fact that the blockage was accomplished with phase angles which, when translated to feedback delays, were on the order of 0.7 msec., suggestively close to the 0.6 msec. feedback delay time of stutterers.

Would it not be fascinating to discover whether young stutterers differ from young normal speakers by similar interaural feedback delay disparities? Would it not also be fascinating to discover whether severity of their disfluent blockages varied with the size of their feedback delays? If these connections do exist, then might you not suspect with some conviction that the blockage mechanism is triggered when the critical feedback delay time, whatever it might turn out to be in children and adults, is reached? And if this is the case, may we not have narrowed our search for trigger conditions down to those that affect feedback delay, especially in ranges that control periodicity of fundamental frequency?

What better place to start than with articulatory rate and communicative pressure? Both conditions are known to affect frequency of stuttering. What is not known is why. Stromsta found that the feedback delay necessary to block phonation varied from one breath supply to the next. This could be related to why stutterers do not block on every syllable. Could it be that blocks only occur when a concatenation of such factors as communicative stress, speech fears, and linguistic combinations affect feedback delay to bring it to the trigger condition for a particular fundamental frequency of a particular sound in a particular breath group?

If the answers to these questions confirm my suspicions, then the answer to the question for which you hired me may be before us. Might not the reason why three-fourths of the children who are thought to stutter outgrow it be that their normal feedback delay times are not as close to critical trigger times as are those of children who become chronic stutterers? Occasionally, they might hit a trigger condition and become stuck, but if feedback delay times are affected by frustration and apprehension, then moments of stuttering would be infrequent enough that they would not snowball into full scale stuttering. Another possibility is that critical trigger times and feedback delay times change with age.

A part of the answer to your recovery question probably also lies in your method of defining stuttering. In all likelihood, some — perhaps many — of your stutterers were never stutterers at all. If you accept my proposition, then repetitions, prolongations, and hesitations are not stuttering unless they occur involuntarily. But the listener cannot make this determination with certainty. Yet, it is the listener who makes the judgment of stuttering. This may be the price you must pay for verifiable observation.

Your President of STUFF has asked me to include my thoughts about clinical implications of this analysis. First, two inferences about early detection of incipient chronic stuttering. The least speculative one is that the children who are at high risk of becoming severe stutterers are those who manifest severe blockage at onset. Until you perform longitudinal studies with direct observation of speech performance, this inference will remain a hypothesis, but it seems reasonably safe.

My other inference is more speculative because it hinges on verification of a casual connection between feedback delay times and critical delay times that trigger stuttering. If the connection is good, then it should be possible to determine children at risk of stuttering, possibly even prelinguistic infants, by measuring their feedback delay times. I understand your profession has developed conditioning methods for detecting hearing loss in infants. Surely you could adapt these to the necessary tests of auditory feedback time.

Finally, I can offer you two thoughts about therapy. One is that both of your major approaches to treatment are effective. The fact that you can gain reasonably good control of stuttering by reducing fear of blockage of speech speaks to the power of apprehension as a trigger condition of stuttering. Similarly, your ability to establish fluency with rate and air flow techniques gives equal evidence that these are also trigger conditions. You will have to determine by your own devices which of these approaches is preferable.

My other thought hinges, as before, on the role of feedback delay in stuttering. If it is critical, then the possibility may be within reach of a prosthetic device that could shorten delay times of children at risk — as well as of confirmed stutterers — that would free them of blockage.

I have done as much for you as I can. If nothing else, I hope I have helped you to distinguish between what the stutterer fears about stuttering from what objective observers may choose to call stuttering. This distinction will make a more profound difference in what you determine to be the nature of stuttering than it probably will in how you go about treating it. For your information, I shall enter your commission in my records as The Case of The Missing Block. Your work is cut out for you. Now, on behalf of Archie and myself, happy hunting.

REFERENCES

Andrews, G., and Neilson, M. Stuttering: a state of the art seminar. ASHA Convention, 1981.

Bloodstein, O. The development of stuttering: II. Developmental phases. *Journal of Speech and Hearing Disorders*, 1960, *25*, 366-376.

Bloodstein, O. *A Handbook on Stuttering*. Chicago: National Easter Seal Society, 1981.

Brutten, E.; and Shoemaker, E. *The Modification of Stuttering*. Englewood Cliffs, N.J.: Prentice-Hall, 1967.

Curlee, R. Observer agreement on disfluency and stuttering. *Journal of Speech and Hearing Research*, 1981, *24*, 595-600.

Howie, P. Concordance for stuttering in monozygotic and dizygotic twin pairs. *Journal of Speech and Hearing Research*, 1981, *24*, 317-321.

Kidd, K. Genetic models of stuttering. *Journal of Fluency Disorders*, 1980, *5*, 187-201.

Stromsta, C. Experimental blockage of phonation by distorted sidetone. *Journal of Speech and Hearing Research*, 1959, *2*, 286-301.

Stromsta, C. A spectrographic study of dysfluencies labeled as stuttering by parents. *De Therapia Vocis et Loquelae, Vol. I*. Societatis Internationalis Logopaediac et Phoniatriae XII Congressus Vindobonae Anno MCMLXV, Acta, August.

Stromsta, C. Interaural phase disparity of stutterers and nonstutterers, *Journal of Speech and Hearing Research*, 1972, *15*, 771-780.

Wingate, M. A standard definition of stuttering. *Journal of Speech and Hearing Disorders,* 1964, *29,* 484-489.

Wingate, M. Stuttering as phonetic transition defect. *Journal of Speech and Hearing Disorders,* 1969, *34,* 107-108.

DISCUSSION

R. Ingham: I guess the model Bill is proposing for us to have a look at is a much more sophisticated servosystem theory. The history of that concept in the field of stuttering has been problematic, principally because it has difficulty in dealing with initial stutterings; that is, stuttering occurs seemingly without interfering feedback, on the very first utterance.

W. Perkins: That's a very good question. Frankly, the thing about the schema I presented that puzzles me most is why DAF that involves 50 to 200 msec. delays, or even less, produces the effect on me that it does. I think what I'm doing sounds very much like stuttering. It certainly seems so to me while I'm going through it. And even though I am role-playing Archie, the blockage is involuntary; it is not fake. Admittedly, my reaction to DAF is peculiar. My speech is more than disrupted; I am blocked. Even stutterers we have tested don't react to DAF with the blockages I do. Now, if you begin to think about the problem in terms of what kind of feedback is necessary to maintain the fundamental frequency of voice, and you think about the ubiquitous characteristics of fundamental frequency (I mean you can't produce any sound or tone that doesn't have a fundamental frequency, and presumably if you're going to maintain any kind of control over the fundamental frequency, you must have some kind of feedback mechanism for it), well, you're dealing then with a frequency rate that is at least 100 Hz. If I'm speaking at 100 Hz., that's 10 msecs. per glottal vibration, but if I'm going to invade and change the feedback time of the single glottal vibration, then I'm down to one msec. or a fraction of a msec., if I'm going to throw it off just a little bit. You throw off the control of the periodicity of the carrier wave, the glottal wave, just enough to make it not correspond with your expectations. So my guess is that the reason I can't get started is that when I generate the first one of those glottal cycles, which is just about within a msec., and I get the wrong delay, the feedback would be altered enough to be unable to proceed. There is nothing in the articulatory tract that I can find that gives evidence of blockage. But we can tinker with breathstream management which involves laryngeal control, and we can turn stuttering on and off. If you normalize the airflow, if you get a laryngeal control task going, such as lipped speech or whispering that frees the air to flow, then all this abnormal articulatory stuff just vanishes. I mean you don't have to do a thing about it. It just vanishes.

G. Riley: We just reviewed 95 stutterers and found that only 35 percent of them involved phonatory arrest. I wondered how your notion fits those children who do not have phonatory arrest, or does it make any difference?

W. Perkins: This is where I'd like to see some longitudinal work. My suspicion would be that the kids that don't have phonatory arrest, judging from Stromsta's study of 38 children, probably are the ones who are going to recover from stuttering.

J. Riley: Is the inference that the delay factor is present in 100 percent of the stutterers?

W. Perkins: That's what I would start out with as an hypothesis. In terms of the children who are going to become chronic stutterers — those that struggle because of their involuntary blockage — I believe you have to ask: "Why are they stuck?" Personally, I'm not persuaded that they learn to become stuck. That really doesn't make much sense to me. If I had to talk under DAF, you'd see a person who had all the anxieties, apprehensions, embarrassments, and everything else that goes with chronic stuttering. Well, I don't, but it is reasonable to hypothesize that such a mechanism exists in children who become stutterers. If you posit a mechanism that is variable enough that trigger conditions can affect the trigger threshold, then you at least have a cohesive explanation that accounts for the group of children who are most likely to find stuttering a life-long problem.

J. Riley: It kind of seems like we're back to the unitary idea of stuttering.

W. Perkins: Well, yes, unless you want to call the other forms of disfluency stuttering. I don't see any evidence that linguistic factors produce the kind of blockage that hangs a stutterer up; that gives him the feeling of being stuck and out of control. If such evidence exists, I have either missed it or haven't been persuaded by it. I know Bloodstein makes quite a case for this. But I've read that case and looked at it as carefully as I could and I'm not persuaded that it really accounts for blockage. It accounts for disfluency. All the forms of disfluency that we identify within a definition of stuttering are accounted for. But my argument is that we have missed the essential element in disfluency if we want to differentiate the clinical condition of stuttering from the condition of normal disfluency.

J. Grinstead: I was just wondering in terms of this essential ingredient for stuttering, what have you done in terms of therapy using that as a framework?

W. Perkins: It poses a real problem in terms of how to identify when the blockage occurs. When it occurs, it's going to be evident in the form of a hesitation, prolongation, or repetition. But the fact that there is a prolongation, hesitation, or repetition doesn't make it stuttering unless it's involuntary, is my argument. The most predictable outcome of treatment, at least with adults, is that they're going to relapse with the kind of treatment we have, which involves controlled speech, controlled fluency. So we decided that what we'd better do is to give them some practice in recovering from relapse. So after they have learned a set of fluency speaking skills, we have them turn off their controls and try to let themselves stutter. What they really hate to do is to let themselves relapse into the condition of being stuck, involuntarily out of control, and we help them learn how to cope with that.

2

Continuity, Fragmentation, and Tension: Hypotheses Applied to Evaluation and Intervention with Preschool Disfluent Children

David Prins
University of Washington, Seattle

The purpose of this chapter is to provide a framework for describing and evaluating disfluent speech that will help to guide decisions concerning intervention with the very young child. The framework is primarily Bloodstein's, based upon his observations of disfluency overlap in the speech of stuttering and normal-speaking children, and the ensuing continuity, tension, and fragmentation hypotheses (Bloodstein, 1981). Bloodstein's ideas will be extended to include possible interactions between tension and fragmentation, expanded interpretations of continuity, and clinical applications for disfluent preschool children.

REVIEW OF BLOODSTEIN

Overlap and Continuity. Wendell Johnson first emphasized the overlapping of speech disfluency types between children believed to be normal speakers and children considered to be stutterers (Johnson, 1959). Although Johnson's data showed considerable difference between normal-speaking and stuttering children in the *frequency distributions* of different disfluency types,[1] he highlighted the fact that no single type of disfluency could be found in one group that was not also present in the other. This finding has been reported often in the literature and was highlighted again recently in the paper by Yairi (1981). Bloodstein, in turn, used this observation as the basis for his continuity hypothesis.

In essence, the continuity hypothesis states that what we regard as stuttering, at least in young children, is simply a more extreme version of the types of disfluencies we find in the speech of normal-speaking children. The fact that there is overlap between all types of disfluencies in children with normal speech and children who stutter is viewed by Bloodstein as a sufficient condition to support this hypothesis (Bloodstein, 1974b).

Fragmentation and Tension. According to Bloodstein, disfluencies originate in a child's speech primarily from an underlying state of doubt or uncertainty about speaking and the attendant threat of speech failure (Bloodstein, 1975). Provocations of this doubt may come from many sources. Initially, they can include such things in the child as articulation and language difficulties, motor control problems, personality characteristics, etc., and their interaction with a multitude of external factors that contribute to communicative stress in the speaking environment (Bloodstein, 1975).

Uncertainty about speaking, as an underlying state, determines how a child goes about the complex task of formulating, organizing, and executing the motor patterns necessary to produce speech. In this manner the uncertainty fosters two underlying (deep) forms of behavioral response: fragmentation and tension. The former results in a piecemeal approach to the task, and the latter results in the use of excessive neuromuscular effort. Each of these response approaches has surface effects on the performance of the complex, serially ordered movements of speech. Fragmentation results primarily in the repetition of fragmented speech/language elements while tension chiefly produces the prolongation of continuant sounds or the extended fixation of stops (prolongations of silence) (Bloodstein, 1974). The fragmentation and tension hypothesis thus provides a framework for explaining the occurrence and distribution of certain disfluency types in the speech of young children. It is important to note,

---

[1]Children labeled 'stutterers' by their parents had distinctly more part-word, sound, and syllable repetitions in their speech than did their normal-speaking counterparts (Johnson, 1959, page 211).

however, that Bloodstein also states that fragmentation may lead to sound prolongations and to silent gaps in speech and that the surface evidence of tension may be heard in speech variations other than simply the prolongation of sound or of silence.

Disfluency Observations — The Young Child. In 1967, Bloodstein began, and others followed, to observe systematically the type and distribution of speech disfluencies occurring in both stuttering and normal-speaking preschool and early-school-age children (Bloodstein, 1974a and b, 1981; Bloodstein and Gantwerk, 1967; Bernstein, 1981; Silverman, 1972; Wall, Starkweather, and Cairns, 1981; Yairi, 1981). The results of these observations have shown consistently that:

1. Whole words are the predominant type of repeated element at this early age.
2. Repetitions occur most frequently on first words of sentences and principal clauses.
3. Pronouns and conjunctions — the short function words — are more frequently spoken disfluently than are the longer content words.

Bloodstein and Gantwerk observed initially (1967) that these disfluency characteristics were clearly in contrast to the characteristics of disfluency in adult stutterers where the tendency is for the repetition of small, part-word or part-syllable fragments, and for the disfluencies to occur on longer, information-carrying words and words that occur later in phrase/clause structure. Subsequently, as a consequence of these observations, Bloodstein (1974b, 1975, 1981; Bloodstein and Grossman, 1981) and others (Bernstein, 1981; Wall, Starkweather, and Cairns, 1981) have conjectured that in the very young child it may initially be uncertainty in symbolic formulation and expression that serves as the principal origin of disfluency. That is, the repetition of whole words at the beginning of utterances suggests, by both fragment size and location, that the child's uncertainty concerns formulation and production of "an identifiable language segment" (Bloodstein, 1974b, page 393). Therefore, it is possible that "developed stuttering has its origin in an early stage of fragmentation of higher order constituents of language" (op. cit. page 389).

To further substantiate his position, Bloodstein (1974b) cites the fact that speech disfluency is most predominant in children at the time of greatest acceleration in the acquisition of adult grammatic transformations, roughly between the ages of two-and-one-half and five years.

How, then, does stuttering as a disorder evolve and take on the disfluency characteristics that we usually see most often in the adult; that is, repetitions of small fragments (part words, syllables, and sounds) with occurrences often on longer, information-carrying words? How do disfluencies change from those that suggest the fragmentation of sentences or word groups to those that suggest the fragmentation of words or syllables? Bloodstein (1974b) explains that words, rather than sentences or phrases, are identifiable by the speaker as repeated elements of expression, and, thereby, over time they become associated with experiences of failure. As a result, they come to engender doubt in the speaker about his ability to utter them, and, thereby, his anticipatory struggle reactions become associated with word cues. Later in this chapter, using Bloodstein's model as a framework, I will offer an additional explanation for the decrease in size of disfluent fragments as stuttering develops.

   Perspective. Bloodstein's tension, fragmentation, and continuity hypotheses provide a model for conceptualizing 1) the determinants of speech disfluency, 2) the evolution of stuttering from so-called normal disfluencies, and 3) the moment of stuttering in the individual with a chronic stuttering disorder. It is important to re-emphasize that fragmentation and tension are offered as the underlying behavioral bases for repetition and prolongation disfluencies in *normal-speaking* as well as stuttering children. Although from a different point of view, these ideas approach the problem of speech disfluency and stuttering in a way that is essentially similar to Zimmerman, Smith, and Hanley (1981). Both approaches provide models to help explain selected kinds of disfluencies in all speakers. Both leave room for ambiguity in categorizing any observable act of disfluency as "stuttering" or "normal," and both permit many intra- and interpersonal factors to contribute to the emergence of a fluency disorder.

EXTENSIONS OF BLOODSTEIN'S MODEL

Figure 2-1 shows Bloodstein's model with modifications 1) To illustrate what I believe are important relations among deep and surface aspects; and 2) To show "frustration" as an underlying interactive component that contributes to stuttering's development from so-called normal speech disfluencies into a chronic disorder.

   In the figure, the solid lines show the principal interactions described by Bloodstein. For example, uncertainty about speaking leads to fragmented and tense approaches to the task that are evidenced in repetitions, sound prolongations, and articulatory fixations in the surface structure of speech. The broken lines — in some cases suggested, but not made explicit by Bloodstein — show interactions between surface speech disfluencies and frustration (1); between frustration and other deep components of the model (2); and between tension and the surface characteristics of sound prolongation/articulatory fixation and speech repetition (3).

   The model illustrates that frustration results from the disfluencies that are a part of, but also serve to thwart, communication (1). Indirectly,

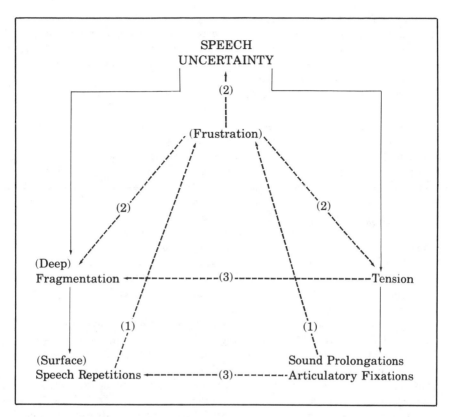

Figure 2-1. Speech disfluency model (after Bloodstein).

frustration then contributes to the growth of uncertainty and, thereby, also indirectly, contributes to fragmentation (2). More importantly, frustation exacerbates tension (2) through its tendency to induce both aggressive and regressive reactions (Yates, 1962), effects of frustration that are extraordinarily significant in the young child from two to four years of age.

The arrows labeled (3) in the diagram illustrate how tension could indirectly affect the characteristics of repetition as a result of its direct effects upon the production of speech sounds. As tension increases, sound prolongations and articulatory structure fixations become more pronounced. [2] As they become more predominant, they, in turn, interfere with the timing of movements necessary for normal syllabic production. As a

---

[2] Articulatory structure here is meant in its broadest sense to include all of the valving mechanisms involved in speech sound production.

consequence, syllables will have a tendency to be interrupted, i.e., fragmented, because of the effect on their production of sound prolongations and articulatory fixations. In this way, increased tension, because of its effects on movement and sound production, helps serve to reduce the size of the speech fragments that are repeated.

The interaction described above expands Bloodstein's notion of continuity by applying the term also to changes in the topography of repetition disfluencies. From this point of view there is continuity in the well-documented change (Bloodstein, 1960) from whole-word to part-word repetitions as the problem of stuttering develops, and it is determined to a major extent by an increase in underlying tension. In this regard, it is useful to note in Bloodstein's (1974b) later descriptions of disfluent children that, as surface signs of tension become more apparent, the children usually also repeat smaller, part-word fragments.

Whether or not there is a continuum of the kind just suggested remains to be seen. Clearly, however, this possibility suggests something different in the usual pattern of stuttering's development than Van Riper had in mind when he said, "In the beginning was the word — the broken word" (Van Riper, 1971, p. 405). The pattern just described fixes the broken word somewhat later in stuttering's evolutionary chain.

It is certainly not unique to view on a continuum the development of behavioral manifestations of stuttering and to use this approach to assist clinical decision making (Gregory and Hill, 1980). The ideas presented above are different chiefly in the sense that the continuum is viewed as a result of interactions between the so-called deep behavior of tension and the surface characteristics of speech disfluency.

Imparting such importance to the role of tension in the development of stuttering is not unreasonable: tension has long been regarded as a fundamental ingredient in stuttering (Van Riper, 1971); empirical evidence points to its universality as a factorial component of stuttering instances (Prins and Lohr, 1972); and attempts to define stuttering objectively have proven difficult without the inclusion of tension (Wingate, 1976, p. 43).

ISSUES IN EARLY CHILDHOOD INTERVENTION

Concerning intervention and the model just presented, I first want to review generally four basic issues: (1) *whether,* (2) *with whom,* (3) *how to intervene,* and (4) *outcome expectancy,* and then to apply these issues to two preschool children with quite different speech disfluency characteristics.

Whether to intervene. The decision of whether a preschool child is stuttering, or is merely disfluent, should not enter into the decision of whether or not to intervene therapeutically. This is made clear by Bloodstein (1975) and is supported by others who have developed protocols for working with the young child (Gregory and Hill, 1980; Curlee, 1980).

Using the concepts of continuity, fragmentation, and tension, the decision to intervene is based upon the quantity and nature of speech fragmentations, prolongations, and fixations in relation to the evidence of factors that may provoke the child's uncertainty about speaking. As mentioned earlier, these factors may include: language and articulation difficulties, with or without signs of neurological disorder, sources of communicative stress in the home environment, and the personality of the child. Essentially, in determining when to intervene, we are looking for signs along a disfluency continuum that signal, not a discrete onset of disorder, but the emergence of difficulties with fluent speech production that are likely to contribute to the child's frustration in speaking. This is similar to looking for danger signs in the child's speech disfluency, an approach found frequently in the literature (Van Riper, 1971; Curlee, 1980; Gregory and Hill, 1980). The importance of taking this approach (vis-a-vis deciding whether a child is stuttering or not) is that it leads to appropriate early intervention, which maximizes the opportunity of preventing a chronic disorder from developing.

With Whom to Intervene. There is no clear-cut basis for deciding whether to work chiefly with parents or with both the parents and the child. If in doubt, it is wise to err on the side of involving both, since many activities that are done with the child serve primarily to model for parents the kinds of communicative situations that are likely to sustain fluent speech. In general, if a child shows little evidence of tension-related disfluencies, but if persistent repetitions of whole words or longer elements are predominant, it is appropriate to begin working primarily with the parents. On the other hand, persistent evidence of tension-related disfluencies and part-word, or smaller, fragments almost always signals a need to intervene immediately with both parents and child — even if these speech characteristics have not been of long duration.

How to Intervene. The question of how to intervene embraces two major issues: 1) program intensiveness, and 2) procedures and techniques. Whenever disfluency characteristics of the preschool child show substantial evidence of tension (including the overlay of facial and bodily signs of tension) and when repeated fragments are predominantly part-words and smaller, an intensive program (several times per week) should be instituted. A less intensive program, e.g., bi- or tri-weekly, is appropriate if disfluencies are persistent, but there is little evidence of tension in the speech disfluencies, and the repeated fragments are mainly whole words or larger.

Concerning procedures, the model focuses our attention on uncertainty about speaking, and about language formulation and expression in particular, as the source of fragmented and tense approaches to talking. From this viewpoint many of the procedures and techniques of therapy should be directed in the broadest sense toward the alleviation of factors that contribute to the child's doubt about his ability to communicate. It is worth noting that some intrapersonal factors that could contribute may be intractable or modifiable only in the long term by specialized intervention programs or maturation, e.g., neurological deficits, language and speech abnormalities, personality characteristics, etc. There are, however, many other possible contributors to communicative uncertainty that are susceptible to immediate change. These include:

1) *General* sources of environmental stress and uncertainty:
    a. erractic planning and conduct of routine daily activities including meals and bedtime.

    b. activity schedules that create unsettling time pressures.

    c. continuing, unpredictable changes in the makeup of the "family" constellation, including relatives and visitors who sometimes live in the home, parental absences, etc.

    d. behavioral demands the child is unable to meet.

    e. insufficient time spent alone with the child and in attending to his individual needs.

2) *Specific* sources of communicative pressure and uncertainty:
    a. poor listening on the part of parents and family.

    b. parental speech characteristics that are complex, rushed, and impatient.

    c. verbal bombardment by parents including constant verbal "teaching" and questions that demand complex responses on the part of the child.

    d. a competitive speaking environment including — persistently — multiple speakers and listeners.

These general and specific sources that can contribute to uncertainty may become the major targets of the intervention program — not only in relation to work done with parents, but also in relation to work done directly with the child. Concerning the latter, this may mean the use of vastly simplified speaking situations in which the language used is initially rudimentary and can thereby assure the production of fluent speech. These situations serve as models that parents observe, take part in, and later transfer to the home. Their therapeutic use will be described in relation to the case presentations that follow.

Outcome Expectancy. The continuity, tension, and fragmentation hypotheses are useful in gauging improvement in the child's speech fluency and in helping the parents to become aware of positive change. Evidence of decreasing tension in struggle-type responses that accompany articulatory fixations and repetitions is usually quite obvious and is a positive sign that the problem is diminishing in severity, at least in relation to the tension component. Concerning repetitions, however, indices of positive change may be more subtle. Signs that repeated fragments are becoming larger in size, are occurring more on function than content words, and on words at the onset of sentences and clauses can be important clues to positive change. In these examples, the repetitions are becoming more like those expected of all children who are in the process of achieving language mastery, and less like those that are associated with increments in tension, and which characterize the discoordination of confirmed stutterers' speech. Thus, a child who begins with repetitions that are predominantly part-word or smaller in size may be viewed as progressing even if, in situations outside the clinic, the quantity of repetitions remains about the same but the repeated fragments have become predominantly whole-word, or longer, in length. Parents may need help to view this as progress along the disfluency continuum for which the continuity hypothesis provides a model.

When intervening with the disfluent preschool child, the expectancy is for rapid change in the clinic and outside if what you are doing is appropriately affecting the factors that contribute to the problem. This is in marked contrast to the older child and adult where evidence of change outside the clinic may come only after a long period of intervention and the use of transfer hierarchies, etc. The principle of rapid recovery in very young children will be discussed again in relation to case presentations.

SAMPLE CASES

Speech samples from two preschool children are transcribed below. [3] Disfluencies are numbered consecutively in each transcription. Descriptions

---

[3]Speech samples are taken from picture and toy description activities. Transcription markings: -$>$ signifies sound prolongation, unexpected hesitation, or articulatory fixation; ⬆ signifies evidence of facial tension or audible evidence of excessive vocal effort; / / surrounds disfluencies; (UI) denotes unintelligble utterance.

and summary comparisons of the disfluencies are shown in Tables 2-1 and 2-2.

Case 1. K. L., age: 4-9; female.
Speech Sample:

        1   2
/Because, because/ a because uhm, because uhm/ a boy is ...

          3
/I mean, I mean, I mean/ the dog is gettin in **(UI)**.

                   4
/But ah, but ah, but ah, but ah, but ah, but uhm/ other boy sittin on **(UI)**.

     5   6   7   8   9
/But, but/da other boy/dis, dis, dis/uhm/sittin on /uhm/on uhm, on uhm/
(UI).

      10   11
/But ah, but ah/but, but/the other people is standing up.

      12   13
/And, and/and so, and so/is the pig.

  14   15   16   17   18
/Ah/bu->t/but ah/but, but/bu->t ah, but ah/but **(UI)** people ring dum bell.

Case 2. R. P., age: 3-6; male
Speech Sample:

     1   2   3
/Go, go, go/goes in the/---->/trash/---->/can.
                     (gasp)   (gasp)

      4   5   6
(UI) /go->/goes/ra->/right in/--->/here.
         ↑   ↑

  7   8   9   10
/H,h/he/ --->/gets the/--->/trash from the trash/---->/can.
   ↑   ↑   (gasp)

```
   11         12        13    14
/Ah, ah, ah/ I/---->/have/dis, dis/---->/truck.
   ↑         (gasp)              (gasp)


   15          16        17    18      19
/Da, da->/that's/s->tring/to, to/ my/po/police/---->/car.
   ↑          ↑                       (gasp)
```

Table 2-1. Disfluency Description.

Disfluency Type:	Child #1	Child #2
Word/phrase repetition	1, 2, 3, 4, 5, 6, 9, 10 11, 12, 13, 17, 18	13, 17
Part-word, sound repetition		1, 4, 5, 7, 11, 15, 18
Interjection	7, 8, 14, 16	
Revision	3	
Prolonged sound	15, 18	4, 5, 15, 16
Hesitation: articulatory fixation		2, 3, 6, 8 9, 10, 12, 14, 19
Utterance Location:		
Initial words	1, 2, 3, 4, 5, 10, 11, 12, 13, 14, 15, 16, 17, 18	1, 7, 11, 15
Later words	6, 7, 8, 9	2, 3, 4, 5, 6, 8, 9, 10 12, 13, 14, 16, 17, 18, 19
Disfluent parts of speech	conjunctions predominate	principal parts of speech
Persistence:		
Disfluency instances/words	18/44 (41%)	19/28 (68%)
Repetitions/instance	up to 6	up to 3

Table 2-2. Disfluency Summary

	Child #1	Child #2
Size:		
% ≥ whole word repetitions	100%	22%
% ≤ part word repetitions	0%	78%
Tension:		
Sound prolongation		
(% disfluencies)	11%	21%
Hesitation; articulatory fixation		
(% disfluencies)	0%	47%
Facial grimaces; excessive vocal effort		
(% disfluences)	0%	42%
Disfluent Words:		
% function (including pronouns)	94%	21%
% content	6%	79%
Utterance Location:		
% initial words	77%	21%
% other words	23%	79%

Comparisons of the children from Tables 2-1 and 2-2 show marked disfluency contrasts along dimensions related to fragmentation and tension.

Child #1

Fragmentation: predominantly whole word and phrase repetitions.
Utterance location: predominantly at clause/phrase beginnings.
Disfluent words: predominantly function words.
Tension: slight, occasional evidence of sound prolongations with pitch rise.

Child #2

Fragmentation: predominantly part-word/sound repetitions.
Utterance location: distributed throughout phrase/clause structure.
Disfluent words: predominantly content words.
Tension: frequent hesitations, articulatory fixations, and facial grimaces.

Before applying selected intervention issues to the speech disfluency characteristics of the two cases, I should note again that many factors in addition to disfluency characteristics would be taken into account in evaluating and considering intervention programs for these children. These include the factors that can affect uncertainty about speaking summarized earlier in this chapter. It is clear in relation to Child #1, for example, that speech is frequently unintelligible and that there are language formulation difficulties. Riley and Riley will present material in their chapter that includes such factors as a part of the evaluation process. On the other hand, I will restrict my comments concerning intervention issues primarily to the analysis of speech disfluencies in relation to the model presented.

INTERVENTION ISSUES — CASE APPLICATIONS

Whether to intervene. In both cases, I would answer the question of whether to intervene, emphatically "yes." In *Case #1* the need to intervene is clear in relation to the problems of speech intelligibility and language. But setting that aside, I am speaking about the need to intervene in relation to disfluency characteristics, even if there were no signs of language or articulation difficulty. The affirmative decision is based on the fragmentation characteristics, even though there is little evidence of tension. Although the size of the repeated elements and their location is typical of the earliest disfluencies that we expect to see in very young children, their persistence is not. In this case repetitions persist in the simplest of speaking circumstances, with a high degree of frequency per words uttered, and of repetitions per disfluency instance. This intrusion on the flow of speech is likely to be profoundly frustrating and thereby contribute to increasing tension and fragmentation with corresponding changes in fragment size, their word and utterance location, etc. The decision to intervene is not made on the basis of determining whether the child is stuttering or is not. It is based on the fact that the child shows extreme fragmentation of phrase/clause structure in a situation with minimal linguistic demands.

   Case #2 should leave no doubt about intervention. Not only is the evidence of disfluency persistent in a simple speaking task, but repeated fragments are often part-words; they include words that occur later in phrase structure, and there is pronounced evidence of tension in sound prolongations, articulatory fixations, and facial grimaces. In fact, the disfluency characteristics are essentially those of a chronic adult stutterer.

   With Whom and How to Intervene. With *Case #1*, considering only disfluency characteristics, intervention should be nonintensive (every other, to every third or fourth week) and should involve the child to the extent of modeling for parents the types of communicative circumstances that contribute to fluent speech.

   This chapter will not review in detail the activities to be used with parents. However, they should be involved in an active, explicit program of observing their own and their child's speaking and listening, and the daily circumstances in which communication occurs. Protocols should be developed to structure and guide these observations, focused particularly on:

    I. Child's Speaking

        Amount of talking in different situations.

        Fluency variations related to time of day, type and number of listeners, language complexity required, urgency, and confusion of situations.

    II. Parents' Speaking

        Rate of speech.

        Complexity of syntax and vocabulary.

        Amount of questions asked.

        Use of "verbal teaching" and explanations.

    III. Parents' Listening

        What they usually do when listening.

        Where they usually look when listening.

        The amount of interruptive listening they and others do.

        The amount of daily time spent "exclusively" in listening.

        The usual amount of one/one vs. one/many speaking-listening situations.

    IV. Daily Routines

        Meals and bedtime, their planning and structure; interactions with factors observed under I, II, and III above.

These observations are structured to allow parents to record and report accurately. The information gained is used to plan specific changes at home that will help to decrease the complexity, uncertainty, and potential for frustation in communicative situations. Some specific suggestions for parental observations and behavior change are reviewed by Johnson (1980). Parental involvement in activities of the type summarized above, when done appropriately and nonthreateningly, also helps to alleviate their anxiety and guilt by giving them an analytic approach to the matter about which they are concerned, and by making them a part of the problem's solution.

Direct work with the child whose speech has disfluency characteristics of the kind shown by *Case #1* is done to model for, and with, parents the kinds of simple, uncomplicated speaking activities that will result in normally fluent speech. Additional comments on such activities will be made in relation to *Case #2*.

Intervention should be immediate and intensive (several times per week) with *Case #2* and should involve both parents and child. In essence, this is an *emergency intervention program*. Evidence of tension and fragmentation in speech is characteristic of that customarily seen in older children and adults who are chronic stutterers. These characteristics, which usually require years to develop, have emerged in a very short time. Parent observational activities of home communication are the same as those summarized concerning *Case #1*. Direct work with the child should involve parents as both observers and participants.

Therapy sessions with the child are structured to control verbal stimulus/response conditions in order to assure sustained periods of fluent speech. Their purpose is twofold: 1) provide a model for parents of the kinds of speaking activities that result in normally fluent speech; activities that parents will participate in during therapy, which will be used selectively at home and will generally set a pattern for simplified communication with their child; and 2) establish and sustain fluent speech for the child for brief periods of time. During these periods the child demonstrates for himself, and attends to, the responses needed for fluent speech production, and he is free of the fluency-inhibiting responses associated with fragmentation and tension that already show signs of becoming stereotyped.

In most instances, carefully controlled, one-word stimulus/response activities will result in fluently uttered words by a child of this age. Such activities, or similar ones (see Shine, 1980), then serve to provide a fluency base for subsequent sessions in which the length and complexity of utterances is increased while the speech fluency criterion is sustained. Ideally, these activities should be entered without verbal explanation and sustained, without interruption, for the session's duration. Reinforcement is is used to gain the child's participation, not to reward him for fluent utterances. Although there seems to be disagreement on this point (Shine, 1980; Costello, 1980), it is my opinion that the responses of fluent speech, assured by the nature of the activity, are powerfully rewarding, and the child's self-gratification is a more significant consequence than a listener's reminder of why the child's responses are desirable.

If factors contributing to speech uncertainty are virtually eliminated in a speaking situation, and if the linguistic demands are greatly simplified, it has been our experience with the preschool child that fluent speech results. Repeating speech fragments, prolonging sounds, fixing articulatory structures, etc., interfere with talking and have no natural appeal. Given response alternatives, and reasonably patient circumstances in which to exercise them, the preschool child will nearly always attend to and use the responses required to produce speech in a way which, for him, requires a minimum of effort and is maximally efficient.

Outcome Expectancy. The expectation for rapid recovery of normally fluent speech is an important difference between working with the young preschool child in comparison with the older child and adult. I do not believe the simplified speaking activities used to sustain fluent responses during therapy sessions for the preschool child are in most cases done as a part of a complex program for establishing, transferring, and generalizing fluent speech. In other words, you are not usually teaching the child a skill or a way of talking that results in fluent speech and that he will acquire by making it a part of his response pattern in a hierarchy of planned therapy activities. Rather, recovery of fluent speech in the very young child is usually spontaneously generalized to outside speaking circumstances. There seems to be substantial agreement on this point (Martin, Kuhl, and Haroldson 1972; Shine 1980; Costello 1980), and a combination of factors may be responsible including: the relatively short duration of the difficulty, its inherently negative consequences for the child, the child's opportunity with your assistance of experiencing and using fluent speech, and your success with the parents in alleviating factors that provoke speech uncertainty. Among the most important of these are improvements in the ways speaking, listening, and communicating generally are done at home. When these improvements are made, in most cases the preschool child will achieve normally fluent speech in a relatively short period of time. This is true even of children with disfluency characteristics as severe as those of Case #2. The behavior of chronic stuttering is self-defeating and unreasonable. Given alternatives, even in the face of failures in coordination that interrupt speech fluency, I believe the young child will almost always find ways of talking that are not stuttered in the manner associated with the chronic speech disorder that carries that label.

SUMMARY

This chapter presents a framework for describing and evaluating speech disfluency in the young preschool child and for making decisions concerning therapeutic intervention. The framework for evaluation relies principally upon observations and hypotheses of Bloodstein, who views stuttering, based upon the continuity hypothesis, as a problem that grows essentially from the exacerbation of normal disfluencies found in the speech of all young children. Bloodstein believes these disfluencies are primarily the evidence of fragmentation and tension in the surface structures of speech.

I have suggested interactions between tension and fragmentation as a useful extension of Bloodstein's ideas in order to explain continuity in the evolution of repetition disfluencies that characterize chronic stuttering. Also, frustration, as a reaction to disfluency, has been added to Bloodstein's model and given a major role in exacerbating the child's tension in speaking.

Certain principles of intervention, although not wholly dependent upon the hypotheses presented, naturally flow from them. Summarized below they include:

1. Intervene whenever there is persistent evidence of speech repetitions (regardless of the size of the repeated elements) or prolongations of

sound or silence that are apt to result in the child's speech frustration. The decision to intervene should not be dependent upon a decision concerning whether or not a child is stuttering or whether his speech could or could not be considered "normal."

2. Intervene intensively (several times per week) whenever there is persistent evidence of tension during speech, as revealed in the characteristics of disfluencies or in other associated speech characteristics.

3. Focus the intervention program on communication in its broadest sense: on language simplification, on the home environment, and factors that can be changed in that environment to alleviate the child's uncertainty about speaking.

4. Work directly with the child in simplified communicative situations that control linguistic stimulus/response parameters, involve parents as observers and participants, sustain fluent speech, and serve as models for parental use at home.

5. Realize that with the preschool child you usually are not (as you are with most older children and adult stutterers) teaching skills through a carefully sequenced program that will help assure speech fluency. Rather, you are enabling circumstances to occur that reduce the complexity and uncertainty of communication and thereby allow the child to respond with the speech fluency of which he is capable. Whatever his capability in this regard, it will be sufficient in most cases to prevent the development of the behavior we describe as chronic stuttering.

6. Realize that some factors that contribute to uncertainty in speaking may not be subject to immediate change through intervention: e.g., language and articulation difficulties, sensory-motor limitations, etc. To the extent that these factors contribute, the need will probably be increased to simplify communicative circumstances and demands at home.

7. Expect a rapid, spontaneously generalized improvement in speech fluency when factors that provoke communicative uncertainty in the home environment are being effectively altered.

REFERENCES

Bernstein, N. Are there constraints on childhood disfluency? *Journal of Fluency Disorders,* 1981, *6*(4), 341-350.

Bloodstein, O. Continuity, overlap, and ambiguity in stuttering: a reaction to MacDonald and Martin. *Journal of Speech and Hearing Research,* 1974a, *17*(4), 748.

Bloodstein, O. The rules of early stuttering. *Journal of Speech and Hearing Disorders,* 1974b, *39*, 379-394.

Bloodstein, O. Stuttering as tension and fragmentation. In Eisenson (Ed.), *Stuttering, A Second Symposium.* New York: Harper and Row, 1975, 1-96.

Bloodstein, O. *A Handbook on Stuttering.* Chicago, National Easter Seal Society, 1981.

Bloodstein, O., and Gantwerk, B. Grammatical function in relation to stuttering in young children. *Journal of Speech and Hearing Research,* 1967, *10,* 786-789.

Bloodstein, O., and Grossman, M. Early stutterings: Some aspects of their form and distribution. *Journal of Speech and Hearing Research,* 1981, *24*(2), 298-302.

Bloodstein, O. *The Development of Stuttering: I,* changes in nine basic features. *Journal of Speech and Hearing Disorders,* 1960, *25,* 219-38.

Costello, J. Operant conditioning and the treatment of stuttering. *Seminars in Speech, Language, and Hearing.* 1980, *1,*(4), 310-325.

Curlee, R. A case selection strategy for young disfluent children. *Seminars in Speech, Language, and Hearing.* 1980, *1*(4), 277-287.

Gregory, H., and Hill, D. Stuttering therapy for children. *Seminars in Speech, Language, and Hearing.* 1980, *1*(4), 351-363.

Johnson, L. Facilitating parental involvement in therapy of the disfluent child. *Seminars in Speech, Language, and Hearing.* 1980, *1*(4), 301-309.

Johnson, W. *The Onset of Stuttering.* Minneapolis: University of Minnesota Press, 1959.

Martin, R., Kuhl, P., and Haroldson, S. An experimental treatment with two preschool stuttering children. *Journal of Speech and Hearing Research,* 1972, *15*(4), 743-752.

Prins, D., and Lohr, F. Behavioral dimensions of stuttered speech. *Journal of Speech and Hearing Research,* 1972, *15*(1), 61-71.

Shine, R. Direct management of the beginning stutterer. *Seminars in Speech, Language, and Hearing,* 1980, *1*(4), 339-350.

Silverman, E. Preschoolers speech disfluency: Single syllable word repetition. *Percept. Motor Skills,* 1972, *35,* 1002.

Van Riper, C. *The Nature of Stuttering.* Englewood Cliffs, New Jersey: Prentice-Hall, 1971.

Wall, M., Starkweather, W., and Cairns, H. Syntactic influences on stuttering in young child stutterers. *Journal of Fluency Disorders,* 1981, *6*(4), 283-298.

Wingate, M. *Stuttering Therapy and Treatment.* New York: Irving Publishers, Inc., 1976.

Yairi, E. Disfluencies of normally speaking two year old children. *Journal of Speech and Hearing Research,* 1981, *24,* 490-495.

Yates, A. *Frustration and Conflict.* New York: John Wiley and Sons, 1962.

Zimmerman, G., Smith, A., Hanley, J. Stuttering: In need of a unifying conceptual framework. *Journal of Speech and Hearing Research,* 1981, *24*(1), 25-31.

DISCUSSION

G. Riley Group Question: The first question deals with the basic model itself — Bloodstein's model. Bloodstein presented direct and circumstantial evidence to support his model. Can you identify crucial experiments to add validity to your revisions of the model?

D. Prins: I am relying more on circumstantial evidence than on crucial experiments with children, except for this: There is a body of literature concerning typical reactions to frustration — not speech frustration or communicative frustration specifically — but frustration from other sources. The typical responses to frustration are both regressive and aggressive behavior of which tension would be a component. What moves me to consider the importance of frustration and tension are my observations, and some in the literature, of what happens when the motor activities of 2-to-4-year-old children are thwarted. Their behavior quickly becomes non-adaptive and disintegrated.

R. Ingham Group Question: My group was most concerned about the actual bread-and-butter activity that took place. For instance, what was the protocol that was used with the parent and the child in the case of both of those children?

D. Prins: The activities with the parents would be similar for both cases. Protocols should be developed very carefully to structure parent observations. They should observe the nature of the child's speech — its quantity, its variations in different types of situations, the disfluency and language characteristics. They should observe their own speech: how and when they speak; the complexity of vocabularly; the complexity of language; the degree to which they ask questions, and answer them; the degree to which they instruct. I would also have them spend time focusing on how they listen. What do they do when their child is talking in different situations? How do they listen? Do they look when they listen? They should also observe the family's listening and communication in general. What kind of listening environment is the child living in? Finally, and not least importantly, I would have them observe and describe daily routines of which communication is an integral part. These are vital aspects of the child's socialization, and include, for example, the periods immediately before, during, and after meal times. How are these routines structured? What do the parents do? What is the child like? Another example is bed time, a very important event in the socialization of any child. Observe how it is organized, what kinds of communication go on, and what the characteristics are of the parents' and the child's speech.

A careful format should be laid out to structure and guide parents' written comments. The format will make observations easy to do and provide material to review with the parents. Using information from the observations, I would focus on those things that can be changed to help reduce complexity and uncertainty. I have not seen a case yet where there weren't many things we could profitably change in those areas.

Now let's turn to the child. Generally, I would begin with structured, one-word speaking acitivites. You can call this a graduated-length-of-utterance approach, if you wish. Even with children whose disfluency is as severe as Case #2, such simple speaking activities usually result in fluent utterances that can be sustained for the duration of a session. The parent should observe and take part in these sessions, and these same (or similar) activities should be programmed for use at home.

J. Costello Group Question: Are you saying that, in order for the clinician to intervene, he must make the judgment: "I think this child is going to become troubled by his speech, frustrated by it, which will lead to tension, which will make him stutter more, etc.?" Do you really believe that clinicians have the experience to make those inferential judgments? Or, are you really saying clinicians can make decisions based more on the quantity of disfluencies? Is there really some objective kind of thing that you're responding to? Also, what child do you **not** put in treatment?

D. Prins: Concerning intervention, if I'm in doubt, I'm not willing to wait and see. If I see a sufficient quantity of disfluency (which I've called persistence) in situations that are very simple and uncomplicated, then I would intervene, letting other features of the disfluency help determine how intensively. I can't give a cut-off point in percentage of disfluencies in a given type of speaking situation, but the two cases in my presentation had about 40 percent and 60 percent disfluencies in a very simple task, and that is certainly well above my intervention threshold. When disfluency is that persistent, it is frustrating to the act of speaking. If it is that extreme in this situation, and the parents report similar, or more extreme, disfluencies in more complex situations, then I don't need to observe those situations to know that speech disfluency is a very frustrating experience for that child. The extent of disfluency indicates that the child is not coping adequately with the speaking task. For him — and for whatever reasons — the act of talking is not done smoothly and effortlessly. Under such conditions I would intervene — because the things that will be done will not only aid the child's speech fluency, but will also aid overall communication and adjustment within the family.

W. Perkins Group Question: Our questions relate to how you get adults involved with children. If the parents won't assume the responsibility for the child, then who could we turn to?

D. Prins: I assume with very young children that, in most cases, you have parent concern. Of course, children might come out of a nursery school screening, or from a nursery school teacher referral, and the parents might be uninterested. That makes it a lot harder. If parents were absolutely unwilling to participate, but you felt intervention was necessary, then I would work directly with the child and do the kinds of things I've already talked about for Child #2. I would probably expand the sessions; have more of them to compensate for the parents' absence. Certainly, a nursery school teacher could do some of the speaking activities that otherwise the parents would do at home.

W. Perkins Group Question: Would you comment on how one might use a preschool teacher?

D. Prins: I would try to work in the preschool environment by having the teacher understand exactly what we are trying to do. Try to set up some simple communication activities in the school environment that the teacher or an aide can do; activities that are controlled in their stimulus-response parameters and that have high assurance of fluency.

R. Ingham Group Question: We have a question that really concerns generalization and the immediacy of its effect. The question is: Up to what age do you expect — what I'll term "natural generalization?"

D. Prins: I couldn't set a cut-off age, but this has happened with every preschool stutterer with whom I have had contact. I think the importance of planning on the rapidity of recovery is that it is a measure of how well you're doing. If fluent speech is not generalizing quickly to the outside environment, you're not focusing on the right things. It takes a lot longer in an older child or adult to know whether you're on the right track than it does with a preschool child. If I saw, in a 5-to-6 year old, the symptoms we just reviewed for Case #2, and if these symptoms had been present for two to three years, I would expect to set up a skill development program with hierarchies planned for transfer, etc., whereas I would not expect to do so for the preschool children I've been discussing. In other words, I would not usually expect the degree of "natural generalization" in children above five years of age that I have described for the preschool child.

R. Ingham: Then it's really the duration factor.

D. Prins: Yes. But I don't know the exact time period. I've been talking about work with 2-to-4-year-old children, and I would usually expect "natural generalization" with them, even under the most severe circumstances.

C. Rossi: What time span are you talking about for rapid recovery?

D. Prins: It's going to be variable. I would say it is sometimes overnight or a matter of weeks when you have begun to change the contributing factors. You may ask, "What are those factors?" In my experience, they have been associated with the communication environment at home. For example, helping parents learn to communicate simply, not to bombard their child with complex language and to demand responses; helping them learn to listen and to structure daily routines to reduce their uncertainty.

Now remember, some factors that contribute to disfluency of speech are not changeable over the short term. For example, the child's sensory-motor abilities that support speech production, his language, personality, etc. These may contribute and may be modifiable only over a long period. These are some of the reasons why you could do everything possible to facilitate speech fluency and still wind up with a stuttering adult. That will happen, but I believe that with appropriate early intervention it will be very rare. Chronic stuttering is so totally unreasonable and self-debilitating that a child will not engage in that kind of behavior, most of the time, if given a reasonable alternative.

J. Costello: Child#1 is not unusual to clinicians who see a lot of kids who have language disorders and fluency problems. If you have a child with multiple kinds of communicative disorders, how do you go about deciding which to deal with first, or, do you deal with them concurrently?

D. Prins: Child #1 was really more-or-less unintelligible. If you did not have the text in front of you, you would not have known what she was saying. From that standpoint, I would work with her intensively, and would focus on language. I would do so because that is the really crippling factor to her communication. I would structure simple language response activities, gradually increase their complexity, but be careful to sustain fluency. Within those activities we could work on vocabulary, word selection, phrase structure, etc. It isn't a case of her language needs being in conflict with the disfluency problem at all.

3

Evaluation as a Basis for Intervention

Glyndon D. Riley
California State University, Fullerton

Jeanna Riley
Rileys Speech and Language Institute
Santa Ana, CA

INTRODUCTION

Recently, a 6-year-old boy with moderately severe stuttering was brought to our clinic. The parents were confused because they had been told by their physician that his stuttering was "neurological, he has a synapse problem and will outgrow it by about age eight," but they brought him in anyway. He had been stuttering since age three.

Most parents are told by physicians and popular literature that their children's disfluencies are normal and they will outgrow them. They come to the speech pathologist in spite of what they have been told because they know intuitively that something is wrong, and parents' intuition is usually correct.

The "non-referral" system just described has resulted in several related problems. First, parents blame themselves as they try to follow the traditional instructions to "ignore it or you will make it worse." (For a recent review of the literature on this problem see Shine, 1980.) Second, treatment is postponed for two to five years after the stuttering can be diagnosed as chronic. This delay in initiating treatment is serious because treatment is simpler, briefer, and more effective with preschool children than with school-aged children. We believe that when the underlying oral motor coordination problems, language problems, and self-demanding attitudes are treated, the stuttering behaviors dissipate in 75 percent of 3- and 4-year-olds without direct therapy (Riley and Riley, 1979). With 6-to-8-year-old children, on the other hand, 90 percent need direct intervention for disfluency. Third, the child is more likely to experience serious social punishment during school years if treatment is delayed. When 20 preschoolers from our institute who stuttered were compared with 24 first to third graders who stuttered, only 5 percent of the preschoolers had experienced serious teasing, but 33 percent of the school-aged children had been so teased. Fourth, word avoidance is rare at the preschool level, but common in first to third grade children. In the same group referred to above, 15 percent of the preschoolers compared to 46 percent of the primary-school-aged children had begun using word avoidance to a significant degree. Word avoidance itself can require many hours of treatment and can prevent fluency modification from being effective (Sheehan, 1970; Van Riper, 1972; Starkweather, 1980).

Ideally, every child who exhibits abnormal disfluencies should be seen within a few months of stuttering onset. Then almost all stuttering could be eliminated before the primary school years. Such early intervention introduces the possibility that some children whose stuttering seems chronic, but who will outgrow their stuttering anyway, will be treated during their preschool years. This is not a very strong argument against early intervention, given the social benefits of an early remediation of stuttering as weighed against the possibility of much more complex, lengthy, and costly treatment later on.

The purpose of this chapter is to describe principles and methods of evaluation of young children who stutter, using a component model approach. Treatment goals which emanate from this approach are outlined briefly.

OVERVIEW AND ASSESSMENT PROCEDURES

A thorough analysis of the child's speech, language, attitudes, and communication environment is central to our approach. It is worth the three hours or more required.

The evaluation includes three principle activities:

1. The Parent Interview asks for parent input concerning (a) onset and development of the disfluencies, (b) a description of the disfluencies when at their most severe, (c) an estimate of how severe today's sample is compared to the child's "average" and "most severe" disfluencies, (d) how they and other household members feel about and react to the disfluencies,

(e) how other children react, especially any history of teasing or mimicry, (f) how the child reacts to the disfluencies, including any evidence of frustration at not being able to talk properly, word avoidance, situation avoidance, or distracting physical concomitants.

2. A Conversational Speech Sample is tape recorded. Fifty to 100 utterances are recorded, which for most children means 300 to 600 words. This speech sample is used to assess fluency, articulation, voice, and expressive language. While making the audio tape, an experienced speech pathologist also makes notes which describe the child's stuttering behaviors that are primarily visual, such as silent phonatory arrest, silent articulatory posturing, physical concomitants, and areas of noticeable muscle tension.

3. Specific Tests are administered if the child's stuttering is considered likely to be chronic. The following areas are tested:
  a. hearing
  b. behaviors related to attitudes, emotions, and attention
  c. auditory processing
  d. expressive language
  e. stuttering severity and prediction of chronicity
  f. oral motor cordination
  g. articulation (if indicated from conversational speech)

INTERVENTION LEVEL I: NON-CHRONIC STUTTERING

Data from the parent interview and the conversational speech sample are used in a protocol to decide if the child's disfluencies are abnormal, and, if so, if they are likely to be chronic. We use the **Stuttering Prediction Instrument** (G. Riley, 1981b) to quantify the data and assist in making some of the decisions concerning the types of intervention that seem appropriate.

Some terms need to be defined at this point. Since all children are disfluent, but only a few stutter, we need to define normal disfluencies before describing abnormal ones. To us, normal disfluencies do not call attention to themselves. They stick out like **well** thumbs, unnoticed. We include the following as normal disfluencies:
  1. Whole multisyllable word repetitions.
  2. Repetitions of phrases of two or more words.
  3. Rephrasing or revision of sentences.
  4. Interjections which are otherwise fluent.
  5. Pauses for linguistic purposes or communication effect.
Abnormal disfluencies are defined as follows:
  1. Part-word repetitions in which a sound or syllable (including one-syllable words) is repeated. Two variables are important in evaluating the

severity of repetitions: first, the number of repeated attempts prior to success in saying the target word; second, the amount of abnormalcy in the repeated material when compared to a normal series of syllables; for example, use of the *schwa* vowel instead of the target vowel; abruptly separated articulatory gestures instead of overlapping movements; tension and struggle behaviors.

2. Prolonged vowels when the duration is 1.5 seconds, or longer. The longer a vowel is prolonged, the more abnormal elements (such as pitch rise, vocal fry, etc.) it is likely to contain.

3. Phonatory arrests of .5 seconds, or longer. These arrests include complete blockage and severe constriction of the glottis resulting in silent struggle or audible, nonvowel-like phonation.

4. Articulatory posturing of .5 seconds, or longer. These abnormally long postures include complete blocking and severe constriction, resulting in silent struggle or prolonged consonant-like sounds. The posture may be appropriate for the target word except for duration.

5. Physical concomitants, such as distracting sounds and facial, head, arm, leg, and body movements. Such behaviors as sniffing, clicking sounds, facial grimaces, looking away, clenching fists, are examples of these concomitants.

6. Accessory features, which are behaviors and attitudes not necessarily associated with a moment of stuttering, but are part of the overall communication pattern. Some of these features include:
   a. the child's behaviors which indicate frustration with his ineffective ability to communicate.
   b. avoidance of certain sounds or words.
   c. avoidance of certain speaking situations.

Listener behaviors in reaction to the child's stuttering can be negative and contribute to the overall pattern of abnormality. Examples of these behaviors include interrupting, rushing, criticizing, and teasing. Or, a listener (especially a parent) may simply be over-reactive to the stuttering, delighted with fluent speech, discouraged with every instance of stuttering, etc.

Based on a review of ninety-five children who were considered to be chronic stutterers and twenty children who were considered nonchronic, seven criteria emerged as the most useful in placing the child in Intervention, Level I (nonchronic) (G. Riley, 1981a). These criteria are:
   1. The disfluencies do **not** include phonatory arrests or constructions.
   2. The disfluencies do **not** include articulatory postures which are prolonged for more than one-half second.
   3. The part-word repetitions do **not** exhibit excessive tension, the *schwa* vowel, or abrupt separation of the repeated sounds or syllables.
   4. The frequency of the stuttering is 3 percent or less per 100 words.

If the stuttering events are very mild, higher percentages may be permitted.

5. The child does **not** exhibit distracting behaviors during the stuttering events, such as hitting his leg, facial grimaces, looking away, etc.

6. The child does **not** avoid words or sounds because of fear of stuttering.

7. The child does **not** evidence frustration about failure to talk correctly; for example, giving up speech attempts or asking, "Why can't I talk right?" etc.

Clinical experience and judgment must be used in applying these criteria. Most children who need Level I Intervention will meet all the criteria. However, some will be borderline and hard to diagnose. Most children who stutter have periods of mild stuttering and periods of more severe stuttering. If you are observing a child during a mild period, you will have to rely on the parent's report of what the stuttering is like "at its worst." You will probably want to see the child again when his stuttering is worse.

Level I Intervention includes placement of the child in a Fluency Monitoring Program. Test data, observations, and audio tape recordings are maintained for two years. The parents are instructed to call the clinic if the stuttering gets worse or if they have any questions. A speech pathologist stays in regular contact with the parents by telephoning every three to six months. The criteria for chronicity are re-evaluated, based on the telephone interview. If there is any question, an in-clinic reassessment is indicated. Parent counseling is carried out during three or four sessions. The goals of these sessions are:

1. To insure appropriate reactions to the child's stuttering.

2. To provide a healthy communication environment.

3. To reduce the parents reactions to the child's attempts to manipulate them by stuttering.

INTERVENTION LEVEL II: CHRONIC STUTTERING

Reduction of Underlying and Maintaining Components

For the past fifteen years, researchers who have tried to synthesize knowledge of stuttering have reached the conclusion that it is not a unitary disorder (Beech and Fransella, 1968; Van Riper, 1982; Williams, 1978). At the 1981 ASHA Convention, Gavin Andrews gave what he described as the last "State of the Art" summary. Because, he said, it will be the "State of the Arts (plural)" from now on. Attempts to describe acceptable subgroups have so far not been very successful (Berlin, 1954; Andrews and Harris, 1964; Riley and Riley, 1979; Riley and Riley, 1980; Preus, 1981; Van Riper, 1982). A component model is a logical alternative to subgroups because it allows us to take multivariant approach without establishing mutually exclusive subgroups. Our current model is shown in Figure 3-1.

There are four components which we consider to be neurologic. We mean that the child has some neurologic dysfunction (or at least difference) which predisposes him to develop stuttering. This notion is consistent with recent genetic models (Andrews and Harris, 1964; Kidd, Kidd, and Records, 1978; Kidd, Heimbuch, and Records, 1981) and with twin studies (Howie, 1976; Van Riper, 1982). The neurologic dysfunctions are not severe enough to be of interest to a physician in most cases. The typical differences are subtle and only show up during the complex functions of language reception and expression, the coordination tasks of speech production, and/or attending responses during demanding tasks. Because they are subtle, careful observation is required.

Recently we surveyed 54 children who were enrolled in treatment in our private practice. This is not a random sample because we have a higher than average number of cases whose stuttering is complex or severe, or, children who have failed to improve using traditional treatment. We were conservative in estimating the "neurological components," and used a rating scale of 0-4 as follows: 0 = not present; 1 = possibly present but borderline; 2 = definitely present to a mild or moderate degree; 3 = present to a moderately severe degree; 4 = present to a severe degree. Only ratings of 3 or 4 were counted, and a child with these ratings was considered to be in need of treatment in the involved neurological component. Given these criteria, four children (7.4%) had problems with all four components, five children (9.3%) had problems with three components, 23 children (42.6%) had problems with two components, 21 children (38.9%) had problems with only one component (usually oral-motor discoordination), and only one child (1.9%) had no neurologic components. Reference to Figure 3-1 shows that without regard to the number of components involved, 87 percent of the 54 children had oral-motor discoordination problems (41 percent also had significant dysarticulation for their ages). Thirty-seven percent had attending problems, 28 percent had auditory processing problems, and 30 percent had sentence-formulation problems.

Each of these components, when present, was described in detail and individualized treatment was designed.

Attending Disorders

If the child cannot maintain attention, it is very difficult to carry out any other treatment. Thirty-seven percent of our sample had attending problems, which were observed by the speech pathologist and/or reported by

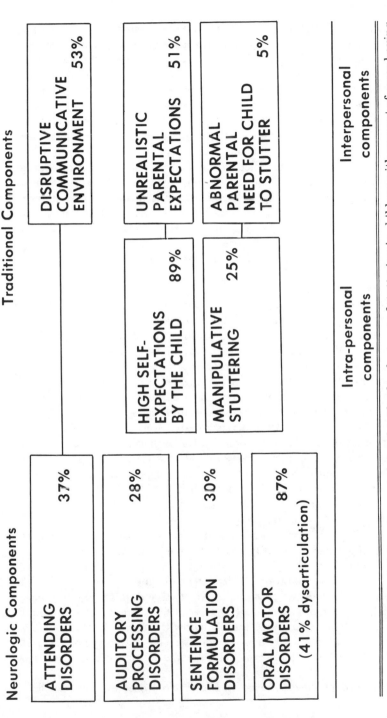

Figure 3-1. A model of nine components related to the development of stuttering in children with percent of cases having each component.

the parents, including (1) **Distractibility:** an unexpected visible or auditory event was reacted to as if it were much brighter or louder than it seemed to others in the room. This often made it impossible for the child to concentrate on any tasks, especially difficult or low-interest tasks; (2) **Hyperactivity:** the child was constantly on the move, reaching for everything in sight, often out of his chair; (3) **Low frustration tolerance:** the child would tend to "blow up" when things did not go as he wanted. These children usually could not tolerate delayed gratification so any reinforcement schedule had to be immediate (usually with primary, positive reinforcers); (4) **Perseveration:** the child failed to change responses to meet the changing requirements of the testing or treatment program. This type of perseveration is more subtle than that seen in a person with acquired aphasia.

Treatment consists of a combination of behavior modification and medication in most cases. The goals are (1) to increase the quality of attending, (2) to increase the attention span, (3) to reduce hyperactivity, (4) to reduce perseveration, and (5) to increase frustration tolerance.

Oral-Motor Discoordination
There is considerable evidence that many people who stutter have difficulty timing the laryngeal, articulatory, and respiratory events which support rapid, accurate syllable production (Perkins, Rudas, Johnson, and Bell, 1976; Adams, 1981; and Conture, 1982). Not all children who stutter, however, have observable oral-motor discoordinations. Among the populations we have studied since 1969, the percentage of stuttering children with this problem has ranged from 61 percent to 87 percent. The lower figure occurred in a population that included public school cases; the higher figure occurred among private-practice clients (See Fig. 3-1).

Every child who exhibits chronic stuttering needs careful assessment of oral motor functioning. We use rapid syllable repetition tasks for this assessment. Currently, we are collecting data for pre- and post-treatment spectrographic anaylsis using the syllables [bʌ, bʌgʌ, pʌ, pʌbi, pʌtʌ, tʌkʌ, pʌtʌkʌ]. Performance observations include:

1. Precision of consonant production.
2. Continuity of performance for 10 repetitions of each syllable set.
3. Voicing errors (especially substitution of the voiced cognate for the voiceless).
4. Syllable order maintained without retraining.
5. Rate of syllable set production. Normative data for children aged six through thirteen are available (Fletcher, 1972). Based on these data, a six-year-old child functioning at one SD below the mean should be able to produce one syllable set 10 times in four seconds, two syllable sets 10 times in seven seconds, and three syllable sets 10 times in thirteen seconds.

To date, our judgments based on the above procedure have not been quantified. A short quantified version is available using only [pʌ], [pʌtʌkʌ], and a tongue laterality task (G. Riley, 1976). Normative data for children aged four through nine are included.

Once it has been established that a child exhibits oral-motor discoordination, we use a systematic syllable training program to improve oral motor skills. We view oral-motor timing as a feed-forward, motor planning process aimed at an acoustic target. There are about 150 muscles that need to be coordinated to initiate and terminate each syllable. In addition, the syllable timing overlaps because of varying transmission times to different muscle groups. Laryngeal timing is the most difficult because the nerves that serve the larynx are so much longer than the nerves that serve the tongue, lips, facial muscles, and velopharyngeal areas. When a child is speaking at a rate of 2 to 3.5 syllables per second, he is executing thousands of neurological events per second, all of which must be precisely timed. Our task is to reprogram the child's "subcortical computer" so that this timing is accomplished with greater accuracy.

We believe that improved oral-motor planning tends to normalize voice onset and termination times, and to improve transitional formants. The child's **fluent speech** will be improved thereby, and the modification of remaining stuttering events will be simplified. Also, we believe that maintenance of treatment gains is likely to be improved because of changes in the child's basic oral-motor system.

Our treatment approach began using the sensory-motor program described by McDonald (1964). It has been modified several times so that now we use a systematic syllable training program which manipulates five variables related to motoric complexity. These variables are (1) number of syllables in the set; (2) number of different vowels used; (3) number of different consonants used; (4) number of unvoiced consonants; and (5) number of consonants between vowels. Performance criteria are the same as those used in testing oral-motor coordination. We start with easy all-voiced syllables in sets of one, two, and three syllables, for example [bi, bʌda, ga da vou]. These sets are practiced in groups of 10 with appropriate reinforcement for success. Second, syllable sets with one unvoiced consonant are introduced [pʌ, dʌta, ka gu ni]. Third, syllable sets with two, then three, unvoiced consonants are used [tutu; pʌ katu]. Fourth, syllable sets are designed with **two consonants between the vowels.** Unvoiced consonants are limited to **one per set** [bʌk, bʌk, bʌk].

Auditory Processing Disorders

Auditory processing refers to the child's ability to receive and manipulate auditory information. Twenty-eight percent of the children had difficulties with this component. It includes not only perceptual considerations, such as retaining an image and making figure-ground distinctions, but also using the auditory information in a more complex manner, such as sorting out the symbolic from the nonmeaningful auditory signals, selecting important cues to syllable and word interpretation, sequencing the input, etc. The behavior of the child who is experiencing difficulty with auditory processing may include such things as:

1. delayed response to the task;
2. apparent need for the task directions to be repeated, clarified, or approached in a different way to break up the erroneous "set";
3. self-corrections as the child responds and then revises his response after he has processed the task requirements more fully.

Several well designed treatment programs are commercially available which are designed to modify the child's receptive language abilities. Wiig and Semel (1980) describe a program in detail and then list some other approaches. Semel (1976) has also developed a separate **Auditory Processing Program.**

Sentence Formulation Disorder

The influence of syntax on stuttering was recently reviewed by Wall, Starkweather, and Cairns (1981). They found stuttering in young children to be significantly more frequent at clause boundaries than at other positions in sentences. This syntax-bound loci of stuttering is consistent with several other studies (Bloodstein, 1974; Hall, 1977; Hayes and Hood, 1978; Kline and Starweather, 1979; Wall, 1980; Bernstein, 1981).

Analysis of our taped speech samples and expressive language testing revealed that 30 percent of the children had difficulty formulating sentences. Specifically, this problem was revealed in (1) word retrieval, (2) short sentences, (3) fragmentary phrases instead of complete sentences, (4) word order difficulties involving word reversals and transpositions, and (5) simplication of utterances, especially the tendency to use only simple verb constructs and to avoid nonpresent tenses and auxiliary forms. Pronouns, prepositions, and conjunctions were often simplified or omitted.

In addition to analysis of the child's speech sample, many commercially available tests can be useful in assessing sentence formulation problems. Sentence repetition ability can be evaluated using the **Carrow Elicited Language Inventory** (1974). The **Bankson Language Screening Test** (1977) scores the child's expressive abilities. The new Clark-Madison **Test of Oral Language** (1981) samples expressive language in several different ways and seems to have excellent clinical usefulness and statistical properties.

Treatment to improve sentence formulation can be devised as it would be for any child with expressive language difficulty. Helpful ideas are found in Hatten, Goman, and Lert, **Emerging Language** (1973) and Wiig and Semel (1980, Chapter 6, Forming sentences: Intervention).

Traditional Components

The remaining five components (See Fig. 3-1) represent our attempt to organize traditional information about children who stutter. The definitions of these components have resulted from clinical observation and parent interviews, as well as from review of pertinent literature. Although difficult to quantify, they are considered maintaining factors of stuttering which, if left untreated, will often interfere with fluency modification or with transfer and maintenance of fluent speech.

Disruptive Communicative Environment

Disruption of the child's attempts to communicate was reported by the parents of 53 percent of our population. The disruptive behaviors included:

1. Conversations that were too rapidly paced;
2. Insufficient silent periods for the child who stutters to organize his thoughts;
3. Interrupting the child during his attempts to communicate;
4. Acting rushed while waiting for the child to respond.

These behaviors were observed via a one-way mirror during family conversations that included siblings. Information was also obtained by parent and child interviews. Such behaviors place the child under pressure, which disrupts the organization of his thoughts and his ability to form sentences.

Improving the communicative environment has long been the subject of traditional treatment of stuttering and, especially, the treatment of young children who stutter. A widely used and helpful booklet is published by the Speech Foundation of America: *If Your Child Stutters: A Guide For Parents* (Ainsworth and Fraser-Gruss, 1977).

Unrealistic Expectations

This component was present at the intrapersonal level in 89 percent of the children in our sample. However, at the interpersonal level only 51 percent of the parents appeared to have unrealistic expectations of their children. Competition was a strong factor within these families. Verbally or attitudinally, parents demanded "perfection" academically, behaviorally, and developmentally.

Since only 51 percent of the parents had unrealistic expectations of the children (compared with 89 percent of the children), the other 38 percent of the children appeared to place themselves under excessive pressure to perform. They compared their efforts with their peers and had a difficult time accepting less than "top" performance. Pleasure expressed by the parents at any success placed undue pressure on the child to maintain excellence. The **Burks Behavior Rating Scale** (Burks, 1969), completed by parents and teachers, was useful in identifying emotional areas. "Ego strength, anxiety, lack of anger control and self blame," were areas related to this component.

When the child demonstrated excessive demands upon himself for fluency, a modification program was used to reduce these demands. First, the child learned to listen to **normal** disfluencies in the speech of others. The child learned to recognize and count these disfluencies in a manner appropriate to his age. Second, the child learned to monitor (in an accepting way) his own normal disfluencies. This change of focus away from the abnormal disfluencies and to the normal disfluencies was usually helpful, and in some cases produced dramatic changes of attitude regarding the need to be fluent. The booklet *If Your Child Stutters* describes parents' reactions to the disfluencies and suggests methods of increasing parental acceptance.

INTERVENTION LEVEL III: CHRONIC STUTTERING

Symptom Modification

Some children do not need Level III Intervention because their stuttering behaviors have dissipated during treatment of the components in Level II. Seventy-five percent of the three- and four-year-old (preschool) children in our sample did **not** need direct fluency modification. By ages five to eight, this figure had dropped to 10 percent, and above age eight all the children needed Level III Intervention. Perhaps at the earlier ages we are assisting "natural processes," which help many children to "outgrow" their stuttering without symptomatic treatment. Neurological development, environmental changes, and individualized coping methods devised by each child are examples of such processes. Component-based treatment may simply take advantage of these processes in very young children who stutter. However, among children five years old and older, stuttering seems to be more firmly established, so that even after the components are treated, the fluency itself needs modification.

After the underlying and maintaining components have been modified to the extent practical in Level II, direct modification of stuttering and its related behaviors is undertaken.

Five basic principles guide our selection of treatment approaches. Any approach included in the program should:

1. be the simplest approach that will handle the problem.
2. be adaptable to any setting and preferably not include expensive equipment.

3. be carefully structured with success criteria well-defined (Prins, 1976).
4. be easily maintained. If, after treatment, the child needs to monitor such things as rate, rhythm, vocalization, or laryngeal coordination, treatment gains will be more difficult to maintain.
5. result in natural-sounding speech, as free as possible from abnormal disfluencies, but not free of normal disfluencies. Also, there should be no rhythm or prolongation artifacts (Runyan and Adams, 1978; Ingham and Packman, 1978; Sacco, 1981).

We have not found any one treatment strategy to meet the needs of all children who stutter. Therefore, we use differentiated treatment approaches depending on the nature of the child's remaining problems as he enters Level III.

Figure 3-2 shows the relationships between the remaining problems and the various treatments. Obviously, a child may have more than one problem, and the usual order of intervention is shown in the figure.

1. Physical Concomitants

The child will often have distracting facial grimaces, head turning, arm or hand movements, foot stamping, unusual nonspeech sounds, etc., associated with the stuttering. Fifty-seven percent of our cases had these behaviors to a severe enough degree to require modification. The child is taught to monitor each behavior and then signal to the clinician his awareness of when it is taking place. The child is reinforced for his awareness. At the same time, the awareness seems to act as a negative reinforcer which extinguishes the physical concomitant. These behaviors are sometimes the most socially penalizing aspect of the stuttering. Since they are more recently conditioned (Starkweather, 1980), they are amenable to direct modification early in treatment. If they extinguish easily, most or all, of them will have been dealt with prior to Level III.

2. Avoidance of Certain Feared Sounds or Words

When a child has developed "word avoidance," this problem must be dealt with first; otherwise, many things presented to the child to improve his fluency will simply be used by him to avoid feared words (Novak, 1975). Recently, Starkweather (1980) described this process and its justification in a learning theory paradigm. The treatment methods have been described extensively by Sheehan (1970) and Van Riper (1972). About 25 percent of our cases demonstrate word avoidance behaviors.

3. Mild to Moderate Part-Word Repetitions and/or Easy Vowel Prolongations

The child's stuttering may be relatively mild and ready for modification.

Figure 3-2. LEVEL III INTERVENTION STRATEGIES: Differential treatment approaches based on problems remaining after Level II intervention.

Problems remaining after Level II therapy.	Simple response contingency	Cognitive modification	Attitude modification	Control complexity of utterance	Airflow management	Approach-avoidance program	Referral to psychotherapist
1. Physical concomitants	②	①					
2. Avoidance of feared words or sounds			①			①	
3. Mild-Moderate PWR or easy vowel prolongation	① RC						
4. Severe PWR, phonatory or articulatory blocks or constriction	③ RC	①	②		③ RC		
5. Syntax-bound stuttering events	②	①		② RC			
6. Severe attitudinal complications			①				②
7. Severe family behavior and attitudes			①				②

ⓧ Circled numbers indicate order of treatment. RC = rate control without DAF.

When a child displays this kind of readiness, a simple response contingency program is usually all that is needed. Costello (1980) and Shine (1980) are among many who have devised useful programs of the type described in detail elsewhere. Twenty-three percent of our cases met the criteria for this treatment approach.

4. Severe Abnormally Repeated Syllables During Part-Word Repetitions, Laryngeal Level Blockage or Constriction, or Articulatory Level Blockage or Constriction

These problems are referred to by Adams (1977) as "Difficulty in starting and/or sustaining voice or air flow for speech." They characterized, to a moderate-to-severe degree, 77 percent of the children in our sample. When present, a carefully planned, individualized, air-flow management program is required. Conture (1982) has described a program which seems similar to what we have been trying to do. He uses analogies and teaching methods to accomplish an understanding by the child of how the voice/air flow is being blocked at the lips, oral cavity, or laryngeal levels. He then trains the child to feel the tensions associated with these blockages or constrictions. Only after the cognitive goals have been reached does he help the child modify these blocks. The modification part could readily be designed into a response contingency program. We agree with Adams (1980) that the modification should be tailored to those aspects of air-flow with which the child is experiencing difficulty.

5. Syntax Bound Stuttering Events

During Level II Intervention, 30 percent of our children needed treatment to improve sentence formulation. Even after this training, some of them continued to stutter more during longer or more complex sentences than during short, simple ones. This distribution continued in a few children even after air-flow management had been improved. That is, they could employ their air-flow techniques better in simple responses than in more complex ones. When this distribution was noted, we employed response-contingency programs which use sentence length and complexity as its variables. Ryan's "Gradual Increase in Length and Complexity of Utterance" (GILCU) program (1974) was designed to accomplish this purpose. To some extent, Costello's program (1980) and Shine's program (1980) also employ utterance length (and complexity, by implication) as variables.

6. Severe Attitudinal Complications

Direct modification of fluency cannot be postponed until all of the child's emotional problems have been eliminated. So, even though attitude modification was employed in Level II treatment, we sometimes encounter children who progress slowly in fluency modification because of remaining attitudinal difficulties. The child may be getting secondary gains such as control of a parent or special attention. In some children, the stuttering has become an excuse for other areas of perceived failure, and giving it up may require the child to reconstruct his entire ego defense mechanism. Sometimes the emotional problems are beyond the competence of a speech pathologist, and the client needs to be referred to a psychotherapist. When resistance to such a referral is encountered, the clinician needs to listen carefully and be sensitive to the stated and implied reasons for it. Some of our more dramatic failures have occurred at this point in the treatment process.

7. Severe Family Behaviors or Attitudes

Once in a while (about 5 percent in our sample), you may encounter a parent or grandparent whose own emotional problems do not permit the child to let go of his stuttering. These cases are very difficult to handle. Extreme neurotic, or even psychotic, conditions may cause a family member to resist or sabotage any successful treatment. We are glad these types of cases are few because they very quickly test the limits of our professional competence and personal ego strength.

Specialized Treatment Techniques

Specialized treatment approaches may be added to the model described above so long as basic principles are not violated. One popular method of attaining rate control, for example, is by using delayed auditory feedback (DAF). We did not find DAF very useful with children. Most children could learn "slow motion speech" when modeled by the clinician.

Another special technique involves spectrographic analysis and feedback to train the child to produce syllables with normal voice onset, duration, and termination characteristics (Webster, 1980). Our program uses systematic syllable training prior to direct fluency-modification to attempt to accomplish similar goals. The stuttering problems are then modified, using airflow-management modification as described above.

Biofeedback using EMG has been reported to be effective in reducing muscle tension in adults (Guitar, 1975; Lanyon, 1977; Manschreck, Kalotkin, and Jacobson, 1980). We find it useful in the cognitive modification to help children with severe laryngeal or articulatory blocks to recognize the tension just preceding the block itself.

External timing devices such as the metronome seem to serve as a substitute for internal motor-timing and coordination. Therefore, their effects are usually temporary. Also, they are oppositional to the internal timing abilities which we try to achieve for these children.

TREATMENT EFFECTIVENESS

Fifty-four children, ages 3-10 to 12-9, entered our component model study between 1974 and 1978 (Riley and Riley, 1979). Forty-four of the original 54 children who completed the program have been followed post-termination for at least 12 months. Of this group, 37 have been followed for 24 to 48 months. The remaining 7 children moved away and/or could not be located.

Eleven children (in addition to the 54) were placed in Intervention Level I. After 18 to 48 months, ten of the children no longer stuttered. One is stuttering slightly more than when entering the program and may need to be placed in Level II.

FOLLOW-UP PROCEDURES

All follow-up was done by telephone calls which were followed, when necessary, by in-clinic evaluations. The parents and teachers were asked if the child exhibited any stuttering behaviors at all. If they did, the criteria described at the bottom of Table 3-1 were read to them, and they made the judgment of "Mild" (score 1) or "Significant" (score 2 or 3). All children with inconsistent reports, and all who were considered to have "significant" stuttering, were evaluated and rated by a staff clinician and the audio tape was reviewed and rated by the authors. The ratings were highly reliable with the few differences being resolved in conferences.

TREATMENT RESULTS

As seen in Table 3-1, twelve children improved from a rating of 1 (mild residual stuttering) to a rating of 0 (stutter free) during the 12 months following treatment. One child improved from a rating of 2 (significant residual stuttering) to a rating of 1 after one year. One child regressed from 0 to 1. Seven of the children in categories 2 and 3 (only slightly improved from pretreatment baseline) remained in those categories during the 12 months after treatment. Between 12 and 24 months post-treatment, two children have returned to the clinic for six or eight sessions of maintenance treatment. One, who had regressed from a rating of 1 to a rating of 2 was able to reattain his rating of 1. The other regressed from 1 to 3 when he reached age 14, and the additional treatment had no measurable impact on his stuttering.

Overall, children with ratings of 0 or 1 were considered treatment successes; those with ratings of 2, 3, or 4 were considered treatment failures. By this standard, the success percent at treatment termination was 82 percent, one year later 84 percent, and 2 to 4 years later 81 percent.

Table 3-1. Treatment results for 44 children ages 3-0 to 12-9 after completion of a component model-based stuttering treatment program.

Rating	No. and % at term. of treatment n=44		No. and % 12-23 mos. post-term. n=44		No. and % 24-48 mos. post-term. n=37	
0	8	18%	19	43%	16	43%
1	28	64%	18	41%	14	38%
2	5	11%	4	9%	3	8%
3	3	7%	3	7%	4	11%
4	0		0		0	

Rating Criteria:

0 = No stuttering reported at home or at school. Speech sounds normal.

1 = Mild residual stuttering reported at home or school but it is not considered a problem by the child or his listeners. Speech is otherwise considered normal.

2 = Signficiant residual stuttering reported at home or at school. Confirmed by clinic examination.

3 = Stuttering was only slightly improved compared to severity at beginning of treatment.

4 = Stuttering was as severe or more severe after treatment.

CONCLUSION

The concept of stuttering as a multidimensional disorder seems to be one among several reasonable approaches. It is compatible with the view that stuttering occurs when combined factors push an individual over his/her threshold of fluency breakdown. A component model such as the one described in this chapter is an attempt to convert multidimensional theory to clinical practice. This model needs to be refined, and relative priorities and sequencing of treatment methods need better definition. The components themselves may need revision. However, we hope that the key idea can be woven into the fabric of our profession, and that the reduction of components causing a person to cross the threshold of fluency breakdown can become a standard tool available to clinicians who want to use a multidimensional construct.

REFERENCES

Adams, M. A clinical strategy for differentiating the normally non-fluent child and the incipient stutterer. *Journal of Fluency Disorders,* 1977, *2,* 141-148.

Adams, M. The young stutterer: Diagnosis, treatment, and assessment of progress. *Seminars in Speech, Language and Hearing,* 1980, *1,* 289-299.

Adams, M. The speech production abilities of stutterers: Recent, ongoing, and future research. *Journal of Fluency Disorders,* 1981, *6,* 311-326.

Ainsworth, S., and Fraser-Gruss, J. *If Your Child Stutters: A Guide for Parents.* Memphis, Tennessee: Speech Foundation of America, 1977.

Andrews, G., and Harris, M. *The Syndrome of Stuttering.* London: Heinemann Medical Books, 1964.

Andrews, G., and Neilson, M. *Stuttering: A State-of-the-Art Seminar,* ASHA National Convention, Los Angeles, California, 1981.

Bankson, N. *Bankson Language Screening Test.* Baltimore: University Park Press, 1977.

Beech, H. R., and Fransella, F. *Research and Experiment in Stuttering.* New York: Pergamon Press, 1968.

Berlin, A. An exploratory attempt to isolate types of stuttering. Doctoral Dissertation, Northwestern University, 1954.

Bernstein, N. Are their constraints on childhood disfluency? *Journal of Fluency Disorders,* 1981, *6*(4), 341-350.

Bloodstein, O. The rules of early stuttering. *Journal of Speech and Hearing Disorders,* 1974, *39,* 379-393.

Burks, H. *Burks Behavior Rating Scales.* Los Angeles: Western Psychological Services, 1969.

Carrow, E. *Carrow Elicited Language Inventory.* Austin, Texas: Learning Concepts, 1974.

Clark, J., and Madison, C. *Clark-Madison Test of Oral Language.* Tigard, Oregon: C.C. Publications, 1981.

Conture, E. *Stuttering.* Englewood Cliffs, New Jersey: Prentice-Hall, 1982.

Costello, J. Operant conditioning and the treatment of stuttering. *Seminars in Speech, Language and Hearing,* 1980, *1,* 311-325.

Fletcher, S. Time-by-count measurement of diadochokinetic syllable rate. *Journal of Speech and Hearing Research,* 1972, *15,* 763-770.

Guitar, B. Reduction of stuttering frequency using analog electromyographic feedback. *Journal of Speech and Hearing Research,* 1975, *18,* 672-685.

Hall, P. The occurrence of disfluencies in language disordered school age children. *Journal of Speech and Hearing Disorders,* 1977, *42,* 364-376.

Hatten, J., Goman, T., and Lert, C. *Emerging Language.* Westlake Village, California: The Learning Business, 1973.

Hayes, W., and Hood, S. Disfluency changes in children as a function of systematic modification of linguistic complexity. *Journal of Communication Disorders,* 1978, *11,* 79-93.

Howie, P. A twin investigation of the etiology of stuttering. Paper presented at the ASHA Convention, Houston, Texas, November 1976.

Ingham, R., and Packman, A. Perceptual assessment of normalcy of speech following stuttering therapy. *Journal of Speech and Hearing Disorders,* 1978, *21,* 63-73.

Kidd, K., Heimbuch, R., and Records, M. Vertical transmission of susceptibility to stuttering with sex-modified expression. *Proceedings of The National Academy of Science,* 1981, *78,* 606-610.

Kidd, K., Kidd, J., and Records, M. The possible causes of the sex ratio in stuttering and its implications. *Journal of Fluency Disorders,* 1978, *3,* 13-23.

Kline, M., and Starkweather, C. Receptive and expressive language performance in young stutterers. Paper presented at ASHA Convention, Atlanta, Georgia, 1979.

Lanyon, R. Effect of biofeedback-based relaxation on stuttering during reading and spontaneous speech. *Journal of Consulting and Clinical Psychology,* 1977, *45,* 860-866.

McDonald, E. *Articulation Testing and Treatment: A Sensory-Motor Approach.* Pittsburgh, Pennsylvania: Stanwix House, 1964.

Manschreck, T., Kalotkin, M., and Jacobson, A. Utility of electromyographic biological feedback in chronic stuttering: A clinical study with follow-up. *Perceptual Motor Skills,* 1980, *51,* 535-540.

Novak, A. Results of the treatment of severe forms of stuttering in adults. *Folia Phoniatrica,* 1975, *27,* 278-252.

Perkins, W., Rudas, J., Johnson, L., and Bell, J. Stuttering: Discoordination of phonation with articulation and respiration. *Journal of Speech and Hearing Research,* 1976, *19,* 509-522.

Preus, A. *Attempts at Identifying Subgroups of Stutterers.* Oslo, Norway: University of Oslo Press, 1981.

Prins, D. Stutterers' perceptions of therapy improvement and of post-therapy regression: Effects of certain program modifications. *Journal of Speech and Hearing Disorders,* 1976, *41,* 452-463.

Riley, G. *Riley Motor Problems Inventory* (rev.). Los Angeles, California: Western Psychological Services, 1976.

Riley, G. Predicting chronicity among young children who stutter. A short course presented at the ASHA Convention, Los Angeles, California, November, 1981a.

Riley, G. *Stuttering Prediction Instrument.* Tigard, Oregon: C.C. Publication, 1981b.

Riley, G., and Riley, J. A component model for diagnosing and treating children who stutter. *Journal of Fluency Disorders,* 1979, *4,* 279-293.

Riley, G., and Riley, J. Motoric and linguistic variables among children who stutter: A factor analysis. *Journal of Speech and Hearing Disorders,* 1980, *45,* 504-514.

Runyan, C., and Adams, M. Perceptual study of the speech of successfully therapeutized stutterers. *Journal of Fluency Disorders,* 1978, *3,* 25-39.

Ryan, B. *Programmed Therapy for Stuttering in Children and Adults.* Springfield, Illinois: Charles C. Thomas, 1974.

Sacco, P. Characteristics of therapeutically-induced fluency. Technical session presentation, ASHA Convention, Los Angeles, California, 1981.

Semel, E. *Semel Auditory Processing Program.* Chicago, Illinois: Follet Educational Publishing Co., 1976.

Sheehan, J. *Stuttering Research and Therapy.* New York: Harper & Row, 1970.

Shine, R. Direct management of the beginning stutterer. *Seminars in Speech, Language and Hearing,* 1980, *1,* 339-350.

Starkweather, C. A multiprocess behavioral approach to stuttering therapy. *Seminars in Speech, Language and Hearing,* 1980, *1,* 327-337.

Van Riper, C. *Treatment of Stuttering.* Englewood Cliffs, New Jersey: Prentice-Hall, 1972.

Van Riper, C. *Nature of Stuttering* (2nd ed.). Englewood Cliffs, New Jersey: Prentice-Hall, 1982.

Wall, M. A comparison of syntax in young stutterers and non-stutterers. *Journal of Fluency Disorders,* 1980, *5,* 321-326.

Wall, M., Starkweather, C., and Cairns, H. Syntactic influences on stuttering in young child stutterers. *Journal of Fluency Disorders,* 1981, *6,* 283-298.

Webster, R. Evolution of a target-based behavioral therapy for stuttering. *Journal of Fluency Disorders,* 1980, *5,* 303-320.

Wiig, E., and Semel, E. *Language Assessment and Intervention for the Learning Disabled.* Columbus, Ohio: Charles E. Merrill Publishing Co., 1980.

Williams, D. The problem of stuttering. In F. Darley and D. Spriestersbach, (eds.), *Diagnostic Methods in Speech Pathology.* New York: Harper and Row, 1978.

DISCUSSION

D. Prins Group Question: Our series of questions all concern Level II intervention. Is Level II intervention done without Level III? If so, for how long? Or are they done together, simultaneously? How often was Level II sufficient if it was started alone? Is it sufficient so that people never go to Level III? And are Level II components worked on in any order?

G. Riley: It's not unusual for very young children who go into Level II, not to have to go into Level III. Only 25 percent of the 3- and 4-year-olds needed Level III intervention after Level II. As they got older — that is the 5-8 group — 10 percent did not need Level III. All of the 9-12 group needed Level III after Level II.

The next part asked when you do things. Except for physical concomitants and avoidance therapy, we never began Level III therapy during Level II. We could start avoidance therapy earlier if that seemed to be a major problem. Physical concomitants can be worked on at any time and quite often we would work on them when the child first came into the clinic because that might be the most socially penalizing part of his problem. We do as much as we can with the speech mechanism behavior before we enter into the management of abnormal disfluencies. And that's of course a part of the theory; that is, we're changing the mechanism from the inside out. Instead of shaping the product, we're changing the producer. It would go against the theory to start shaping the product before you do as much as you can to change production, for example.

Now the next part of the question dealt with the order in which we work. We've never been able to set this in a nice straight pattern that seems to work for every child. Attending comes first. That part is easy because if you can't get the child's attention, you can't do anything else. The oral-motor discoordination treatment is usually started right away because it tends to be a fairly lengthy task. Of the nine components, it's probably one of the most basic changes. The environmental components are treated in parallel with the neurologic ones. We're working on them in parent conferencing. A lot goes on during the sessions with the parents — explanations of what we're doing with the child, explanations of any homework-type assignments, and carry-over.

When it comes to attitude changes, like the child's sense of worth, the child's sense of anxiety, "Have I got to do it right?", "If I don't do it right, I'm a bad boy," — those things do not program well. You can write a fairly good goal but it's hard to write the specific objectives and, especially, a time line. We probe fluency at the beginning of almost every session. Sometimes the *content* of the probe opens up something we may spend half-an-hour on even though it's not in our therapy plan, because it is an opportunity to work with the child's attitude.

Now, the parents. We don't think it makes much difference if a parent is strict or permissive. All that does is establish how far out the lines will be drawn. Eventually, there's something the child wants to do that he can't do, otherwise you have anarchy. So, whether you consider yourself a strict parent, meaning rather close-together lines, or permissive parent, meaning the child's play area is bigger, he still has a line that he can't cross. And that's when books like "Dare to Discipline," "How to Rear Your Children," etc., start coming into play. We certainly have assigned things for the parents to read and then have information sessions learning about how to rear children. We don't assume that we know much about how a parent ought to rear a child. But we do know some things that we **don't** want to happen. We ask the parent to try to prevent these things from happening, specifically, the child using stuttering to manipulate, and certain things in the home environment which deny the child a chance to communicate.

J. Costello Group Question: I think the major questions that we were interested in were the references that would describe your test battery. Also, people were particularly interested in your measures of auditory processing. You might want to describe that part of your battery.

G. Riley: We turned in two articles about the same time. The *Journal of Speech and Hearing Disorders* article was a factor analysis of the motoric and linguistic variables. It describes 19 variables and how each of these variables was defined. The other one was in the *Journal of Fluency Disorders* in December, 1979. It describes the measurements with regard to each component. We don't think it's very important which instrument you use for auditory processing measurement. For clinical purposes, you can make a very good judgment of it just by writing down the word delays, perseveration, self-correction, repeated cues, and repeated instruction that may be needed. Then give the child a game, something that requires a little bit of instruction, and see how many times he catches on right away, how many times he delays, how many times he needs another cue, how many times he needs a repetition, etc.

J. Riley: I'd like to add a comment. You could use the *Porch Index of Communicative Ability in Children* (PICAC) for auditory processing if you wanted an objective number. It's scored on a 1 through 15 scale instead of plus, minus. And cued response, repetitive response, delayed response, all of those have specific numbers. You can look through and see how many 12s, and how many 13s, how many 9s, etc. And you can count very quickly the number of times the child had to go through that kind of processing.

W. Perkins Group Question: We had a three-part question. The first was: How did you select the tasks to determine your components? Now, we realize that the components were factored out, but they were factored out from the tasks you selected. So you must have had some preconception of what you were looking for before you searched for the components. The second was, How do you use this component analysis in clinical decision making? You've got percentages that fall out from your factor analysis based on your group performance. But how do you use that in clinical decision making for the treatment of the individual case? The last question is that we'd like to know a bit more about what you do in treating neurologic components.

G. Riley: I'll try to sketch it. Initially, we just took every test that we could think of, including some things that we made up. From 56 variables we finally got down to 19. Then we tried to stay with tasks that had better statistical characteristics and were more widely used in research. We had collected files of data that showed a language group, an oral motor group, and emotional group, a developmental group. We had those four groups and they kept expanding into different subgroups. There were some biases built into the choice, but that's how it came about.

W. Perkins: Were the biases there before you selected the first 56?

G. Riley: The biases were there. We expected that there would be some language problems and we expected to find some motor problems. At first, we started finding about two-thirds of our children with oral-motor problems, and nobody else was reporting that too much. We went through a period of doubt. Maybe we were finding things that weren't there. But then, thanks to your work and others, it became acceptable to have found oral-motor discoordination problems, and that helped considerably.

W. Perkins: How do you use these component analyses for clinical decision making for the individual case?

G. Riley: The percentages in the tables I presented represent the number of children that demonstrated that particular thing to a clinically significant level. With each child we make out a chart of components. Then we look at what strengths we can build on. We resolve in conference any differences we have about the levels and the scoring. We staff the child and ask, "Where is the handle?" It's an individual kind of decision for each child.

W. Perkins: Could you speak to whatever it is you think is effective in Level II?

G. Riley: The most important thing we think is the syllable training program; the systematic syllable training and the sentence formation.

W. Perkins: Could you give us just a sample of what you do in that?

G. Riley: It's very simple. We have 5 variables. We have the number of syllables in the syllable set, like /ba/, /baba/, /bababa/. We have the number of different consonants. (In that particular one there was only one consonant, "b," although it was used over and over again. If I did /baga/, that would have two consonants.) We have the number of vowels. (/bagi/ would be two vowels and two consonants.) We also use the number of unvoiced elements, even if it's the same consonant; /pʌ, pʌ, pʌ/, has three unvoiced elements per training unit. And, finally, we use the number of consonants between vowels, so if I have /pak bi/, the "k" and "b" are between vowels. We think that moves from simple to complex.

J. Costello: And if the child stutters, you just ignore it?

G. Riley: Yes, but stuttering is rare. When children stutter on the presented syllables so that the training breaks down, we have to work on some other approaches. Sometimes we can go for all VC units instead of CV ones. For example, they don't stutter on /ak, ak, ak/, but they do on /ka, ka, ka/. I'd say only one or two out of the 54 would have given us any trouble that way.

S. MacFarlane: How many sessions would you have with a child?

G. Riley: The overall average, for the total program for a three-to-five-year-old, is 48 hours. For a six-to-eight-year-old, it's around 64 hours. I don't have the numbers above that. We do not find intensive work to be as useful as spreading it out because we think there's some incubation involved. There's some home practice involved that's important. Now the syllable training part of the program probably varies anywhere from 12 to 24 hours. The average is 16.

R. Ingham Group Question: I really do think that you have covered most of the questions that were raised in our group. But I'd like to pass a comment. I'm most admiring of the tremendous amount of effort that you've put into what is essentially a format for a private practice. My suspicion is that this sort of system, and I don't mean this disparagingly, is a commercially viable sequence of procedures that can be managed within a typical clinical arrangement. You start children in a very simple procedure, such as the ELU procedure, and move to much more complex and demanding procedures as a consequence of any difficulties that you find as you proceed. I don't know whether there's even a question there, it's just an admiring comment for what I perceive you've developed. And thank you for sharing it.

4

Current Behavioral Treatments for Children

Janis M. Costello
University of California, Santa Barbara

There are some things you should know about me before I begin. I am a clinician. I enjoy doing clinical work, especially with very young children who stutter. I like the kids (as long as they are not mine!), and I genuinely enjoy the challenge of helping them change their speaking for the better. It makes me feel that I've put in a worthwhile day's work when I know that someone's speech (and maybe his or her whole life) is going to be better because of the time we've spent together. I am also a scientist. I like data as much as I like young stuttering children. And a good deal of the satisfaction I get from the clinical work I do is because I know for sure when I've been successful (because the data tell me); I generally understand what it was that I did that produced positive effects in my client's speech (because the data tell me); and I can produce those effects again with the next client. That's part of what being a scientist is. The treatment that I design for each client is based upon theory, upon laboratory data generated by myself and others, and upon my own past clinical experience which is bolstered by online treatment data and experimental manipulations made in the actual treatment setting and during actual treatment. My laboratory is my clinic is my laboratory. Now that's not to say that all of the stuttering treatment I have ever designed and delivered has been successful. But it is to say that when it is not successful, I know it, not just because my client keeps stuttering, but because I have precise data about how much he or she is stuttering and about exactly how stuttering and fluency change in response to different things I try. All I'm doing as a clinician-researcher is using my knowledge of stuttering and my powers of observation in careful and systematic ways. That's something all of us can do.

It is my belief (Costello, 1979) that a line separating clinicians and researchers should not be drawn. That is, as a clinician one must accept the responsibility of acting as carefully and with as much rigor as a scientist. Clinicians can have a powerful influence on their clients and that influence should be taken seriously. Clinicians have the responsibility to understand their own clinical techniques — why they work, what about them works, and that they *do* work for the benefit of the client. Therefore, all of us who are clinicians must accept the responsibility of continually assessing the quality of what we're doing in our own treatment. Best of all, that's not difficult to do. It's even fun. More about that as we progress.

Another thing that should be known about me before we begin is the basic premise from which I operate where stuttering children are concerned. Stuttering in young children (even in very young children) can be successfully treated, should be treated, must be treated if we, as clinicians, are to perform ethically and adequately. Young children who stutter are not to be frightened of, are not to be wary of, and are, in fact, some of the most delightful clients you will ever see. Further, for the most part, their stuttering is not particularly difficult to treat. If a child is old enough to use connected speech and to be noted as a stutterer (the youngest we've seen was just over age two), then that child is eligible for stuttering treatment (targeted directly at stuttering and fluent utterances).

Now that you know some things about me, let me tell you some things that I know about you. I know that most of you feel (probably accurately) that your education in the area of stuttering treatment is minimal, at best. You probably know a lot about theories of stuttering, but very little about its treatment. I also know that most of you do not have a lot of stutterers in your caseloads, so you don't have much occasion to read the literature on stuttering or to become familiar with the ins and outs of stuttering and stutterers. These two factors together, lack of an academic background in which you feel confident where stuttering is concerned, and lack of practice in dealing with clients who stutter — especially the little ones, probably make you a bit nervous about working with young children who stutter. Further, the (nonexperimental) literature is replete with theories of stuttering that make us exceedingly cautious with such children for fear we will heighten their awareness of their stuttering or do any of a myriad of other things that might make their stuttering worse instead of better. And since we don't clearly understand what makes them stutter in the first place, it's difficult to guard against doing something that might precipitate a turn for the worse. And so we're glad for the opportunity to stay away from stuttering clients, yet we know that as clinicians we can't do that.

If these sentences express some of your feelings and experiences, let me point out to you that you are not at all alone. In 1971, Wingate wrote a wonderful article entitled "The Fear of Stuttering" in which he stated, "I believe that one could develop impressive substantiation for the complaint that most speech clinicians are, in their own way, more afraid of stuttering than many of the stutterers they are called upon to treat" (p. 3). And here we are in 1982, and Wingate's statement is still all too true.

There was also a very interesting article published recently by St. Louis and Lass (1981). They administered a paper-and-pencil inventory called the CATS to freshmen, sophomores, juniors, seniors, masters, and doctoral students in university speech and hearing programs throughout the country. (CATS stands for Clinicians' Attitudes Toward Stuttering Survey, and it was developed by Cooper and presented as an ASHA paper in 1975). Through students' responses on this questionnaire, St. Louis and Lass found that students generally believe that stutterers have serious psychosocial problems, that stutterers do not have physiologic components to their stuttering, that counseling for stutterers and their families is a crucial component to treatment, that there is truth to Johnson's (1967) semantogenesis theory which warns us not to label or draw attention to a child's disfluencies because that will cause stuttering, and that clinicians aren't very competent where the treatment of stuttering is concerned. The data also indicate that these attitudes of speech-language pathology students become more ingrained as their level of education increases. Further, St. Louis and Lass' findings parallel those of Cooper (1975) who studied practicing speech-language clinicians. Cooper summarized his results by saying that speech clinicians are continuing to be influenced by old attitudes that are unsubstantiated by research. St. Louis and Lass found this to be true of students currently being educated, as well. Somehow these rumors about stuttering, what causes it, and how it should be treated continue to be promulgated. It is my hope that what you will have learned by the time you finish reading this book is that conducting direct stuttering treatment with young children is not only possible, it is necessary and highly likely to be successful; and there's no reason in the world why you shouldn't be doing it.

EARLY VIEWS OF STUTTERING TREATMENT FOR YOUNG CHILDREN

Please note that I am talking about the appropriateness of conducting treatment aimed *directly* at the way in which young stuttering children are speaking — at increasing their fluency and decreasing (eliminating) their stuttering. A better-known approach to treatment of the young stutterer (when one is advocated at all) is an indirect approach aimed at the alteration of environmental variables hypothesized to influence the occurrence of stuttering. If you read the literature, and especially if you read the pamphlets that are written as information to parents (Ainsworth, 1975; Ainsworth and Fraser-Gruss, 1981; Cooper, 1979; Johnson, 1967), you will find that authors have been attempting to describe environmental factors that should be targets for treatment in the families of young stutterers. In general, these authors ascribe to the rule that you should be a good parent. There are obviously many ways to do this, but these writers typically suggest being a good listener, making sure the child knows he or she is loved, providing good speech models in terms of articulation, speaking rate, and language complexity. They further suggest that parents should: reduce the amount of punishment in the child's environment, increase the amount of reinforcement, help the child develop an expanded vocabulary. Further, parents should not: let the child get excited, let the siblings interrupt when the child is talking, call attention to the child's disfluencies, demand perfect speech. There are many more of these do's and don't's, but you get the picture. All of the tenets of good parenting are invoked and the responsibility for the child's stuttering is typically placed squarely on the shoulders of the parents. Hence, the responsibility for alleviating the child's problems rests with them as well.

I have three things to say about all of this. First, to my knowledge, there are essentially no data to support any of the above-described contentions. That is, our literature is full of theoretical and philosophical pleas to our logic about environmental variables that could induce stuttering, but basically none of these variables has ever been clearly shown to be functionally related to stuttering. No rigorous experimental evidence exists to demonstrate that the presence or absence of any particular family-environmental variable, or composite of variables, is a functional antecedent to stuttering. For example, if we were to believe that aversive or punishing interactions between a child and his or her parents aggravated (or produced) stuttering, then we would need to see an experiment that demonstrated a high rate of stuttering during interactions that one would describe as negative, and a low rate of stuttering (preferably in the same child) when the environment was arranged so that no negative parent-child interactions occurred. (Actually, an attempt at research on this variable was conducted by Egolf, Shames, Johnson, and Kasprisin-Burrelli in 1972, and by Kasprisin-Burrelli, Egolf, and Shames in 1972, although the experimental design and clarity of the findings in these studies were less than adequate for the demonstration of a causal relationship.)

To me, the issue is ultimately an ethical one. Do we have the right to ask families to rearrange their lives and alter their interactions with one another, and do we have the right to imply to them that the child's stuttering is a by-product of their interactions with him or her, when we do not

know, with any level of empirical confidence, which, if **any,** of a large number of factors are truly related to the child's stuttering? I believe that we do not have this right without convincing and replicated empirical evidence to guide us. Such evidence may eventually exist. When it does, the nature of the treatment I provide stuttering children will change accordingly.

A second issue of concern to me is the likelihood of such treatment really being effective. That is, how well are we able to effect family members' behaviors, anyway? When one is trying to produce change in the family environment, and the treatment/counseling is going on in the clinical environment, one is basically operating through advice and conversation. We try to get reports from the family members about their behavior and the child's; but the accuracy of these reports is always to be questioned, no matter how well meaning the family members may be. For the clinician, it is very difficult to produce behavior change when one doesn't have control over many of the relevant variables that could influence family members, and when one can't reliably observe (let alone measure) the behaviors of interest. This kind of long distance, second-order treatment, aimed at changing family members' behaviors beyond the confines of the clinician's office, seems to me to be a rather distant and imprecise method of affecting change. Further, if we combine this problem with the first problem — that of the clinician not clearly knowing what aspects of the stuttering child's family environment to change, the shaky ground on which this kind of treatment is built becomes even more obvious.

Third, there are a good number of studies (to be described below) that rigorously and empirically demonstrate that direct treatment of stuttering in children is feasible. Further, when we deal directly with the stuttering child and his stuttering and fluent behaviors, we have the opportunity to observe and measure the behaviors of interest and to manipulate treatment variables under our control. Since I believe that altering family members' behaviors — even were some to be shown clearly related to stuttering — is difficult at best, it seems to me that a more suitable strategy for treating stuttering in young children is to directly teach them to produce fluent, nonstuttered speech no matter what is going on in their natural environment.

DIRECT TREATMENT OF STUTTERING
IN YOUNG CHILDREN

Let's turn, then, to a brief review of some of the research directed toward evaluating the effectiveness of direct treatment of stuttering in young children. The research can be divided into two categories: articles that concentrate on the positive reinforcement of fluency, and articles that include the punishment of moments of stuttering. Since stuttering and fluency are essentially reciprocals of one another — a given syllable produced by a speaker is essentially either stuttered or produced fluently — the problem has been addressed from both directions. That is, if treatment produces an increase in fluent utterances, there will necessarily be less stuttering. And the reverse is also true: if treatment is directed at reducing the frequency of stuttering, the talker will necessarily be more fluent (as long as we describe a fluent utterance as one which contains no stuttering — an issue that turns out not to be as simple as it sounds [Adams, 1981; Few and Lingwall, 1972; Hegde, 1978; Ingham and Carroll, 1977; Ingham and Packman, 1978; Metz, Conture, and Caruso, 1979; Starkweather and Myers, 1979; Stephen and Haggard, 1980; Wendahl and Cole, 1961; Zimmerman, 1980]).

The positive reinforcement of fluent utterances. One of the early experimental studies of the reinforcement of fluency in children was accomplished by Shaw and Shrum (1972), although the philosophy was suggested earlier by Bar (1971). Shaw and Shrum treated three male stuttering children who were nine and ten years of age in an ABAB reversal design (Hersen and Barlow, 1976) over four, 20-minute sessions. In the first session, baseline data were collected while the child conversed freely with the clinician. During this time, each child's speech was observed so that a fluency target for treatment could be pinpointed. For two of the children, a fluency duration of 10 seconds (that is, 10 seconds of continuous talking without stuttering) was selected, while five seconds of continuous fluency was the target behavior for the third child. During the baseline session, the number of targeted fluent utterances that occurred was counted for each child. At the beginning of the second session, the child was told of the reinforcement system wherein the clinician would mark off a square on a page of 48 squares every time the child talked without stuttering. Stuttering was then modeled for and practiced by the child. It was explained that when all 48 squares were marked off, the child would earn a backup reinforcer, which he selected at this time. After these instructions and explanations, session two was conducted during which the clinician marked off one square every time the child spoke fluently for the required amount of time. Fluent utterances were observed to increase substantially (and thus stuttering decreased) for all subjects in comparison to baseline. At the beginning of the third session, the clinician explained that now the child would get a square crossed off every time he stuttered, and the clinician modeled stuttering responses and had the child practice them. Essentially, then, in this condition the contingencies were reversed and stuttering, rather than fluency, was reinforced. The data for all three subjects indicated that stuttering returned at least to baseline levels (thus fluent utterances decreased in number) during this condition.

Now you might ask why one would want to reinforce stuttering, of all things. However, this procedure is valuable for two reasons. First, the fact that changes in the frequency of fluent utterances and stuttering coincide with the introduction and removal of the reinforcement contingency serves to indicate that those behavior changes were a function of the experimental manipulation of the independent variable, reinforcement. That is, they didn't happen by accident or for some unknown reason. It is most likely that fluency increased in the first place because it was being reinforced, and that it subsequently returned to baseline levels because it was no longer being reinforced. Further, these data serve to indicate that fluency may be just a "plain old response" like any other response. When it was reinforced, it increased in frequency of occurrence; and when an incompatible response was reinforced (in this case, stuttering), it decreased. These data might lead us to believe that we need no special principles of behavior to describe and understand fluency and stuttering. The principles already well known to behavioral psychology serve quite adequately.

Following the reinforcement of stuttering and the subsequent decrease in fluent utterances in the third session, fluency was once again reinforced in session four, and once again it increased (and stuttering reciprocally decreased). Here we see the effects of the contingencies observed in the second session being replicated, giving us yet more confidence in the findings. Thus Shaw and Shrum were able to demonstrate that reinforcement for fluency (at least when the reinforcement contingencies were combined with instructions) produced clinically significant changes in fluent and stuttered talking in children.

A similar study was conducted by Peters (1977) with two eight-year-old male stutterers in a public school setting. When a predetermined number of tokens had been earned for fluent utterances of a particular length, the child was allowed to bring a friend to the next session (the child-selected reinforcer). The data indicated that stuttering was essentially eliminated in the clinic setting within a time span of three-and-a-half to four months.

A variation of the reinforcement-for-fluency strategy was conducted by Johnson (1980), who taught parents of seven young stuttering children to treat their children's stuttering themselves, in the home setting. Parents were taught to ignore children's talking when it contained moments of stuttering, and to reinforce with attention and interaction those utterances that were fluent. She also asked the parents to speak more slowly to their children because it was her hypothesis that some children who stutter may speak too rapidly and that if the parents slowed down their speech, maybe the children would, too. (Although speaking-rate data did not indicate that these subjects were speaking too rapidly before treatment, they were speaking more slowly during the posttreatment measures.) The data from this study tend to indicate that children's fluency improved over time with this parent-administered treatment wherein parents were instructed to selectively attend only to their child's fluent utterances. However, no data on parent behavior were obtained, so we can't verify that parents actually applied this technique, or that they slowed their speaking rates when communicating with their children. Their anecdotal reports appear to indicate that the parents felt the selective attention for fluency was the more powerful of the two procedures.

The addition of punishment of stuttering. Punishment studies have centered their attention on the stuttering moment, although most of these studies have combined punishment for stuttering with reinforcement for fluency — in my opinion, the only appropriate way to use punishment contingencies (Costello and Ferrer, 1976).

I've always been sorry that Skinner didn't invent a more neutral word than *punishment* to describe this set of procedures. Reinforcement is a rather neutral word. It doesn't necessarily carry a lot of connotations along with it, and we can learn to utilize it appropriately as a precise, scientific, technical term. Punishment, on the other hand, certainly does carry a lot of excess baggage in terms of our previous, nonscientific connotations of the meaning of the word. It connotes anger, physically and psychologically intense and sometimes painful interactions, the things our mothers did to us when we were bad (or when we really didn't deserve it), etc. Punishment is generally thought to be a bad thing. But when one is using the term as a part of the technical terminology of behavioral psychology, punishment simply means attaching a consequence to behavior and observing a subsequent decrease in the frequency of occurrence of that behavior. It doesn't mean using a shock stick on children who stutter. It doesn't mean yelling at a child every time a moment of stuttering occurs. It just means following that moment of stuttering with some kind of feedback — a consequence — that produces a reduction in that behavior. It may be a seemingly neutral consequence. It may be saying "No!" It may be taking a token away. It may be frowning. It may be asking the child to stop talking for a moment, or to slow down, or to repeat the utterance. It may be innocuous, or it may be more intense. The nature of the "punishing" stimulus depends upon the child and what is functional for that particular child.

Some of the stuttering literature would lead us to believe that if you punish stuttering, it increases (e.g., Brutten and Shoemaker, 1967). It doesn't. If a moment of stuttering occurs and is followed swiftly by an effective punishing consequence, the frequency of stuttering will decrease. The early research that first demonstrated this finding, and a comprehensive discussion of punishment issues, is provided in an excellent article by Siegel (1970).

So let's turn now to a review of some of the more recent, clinically oriented research with stuttering children and punishment contingencies. The first study to bravely forge ahead and test the use of punishment contingencies with young children who stuttered was conducted by Martin,

Kuhl, and Haroldson (1972). (It was pretty daring to attempt to punish stuttering in young children in 1972, because the ghost of Wendell Johnson was still hovering over stuttering theory and practice!) Their two subjects were male stutterers aged 3-6 and 4-6. In this ABA withdrawal design (Hersen and Barlow, 1976), each child was engaged in conversation with a puppet named Suzibelle. During the baseline sessions, Suzibelle and the child conversed while the experimenters measured the child's rate of stuttering until it was stable over time. Then, when the experimental treatment was introduced, each time the child stuttered the puppet would briefly stop talking to the child and go limp, and the lights illuminating Suzibelle would go out. As long as the child was talking fluently, he could maintain Suzibelle's attention (reinforcement for fluency); but as soon as a moment of stuttering occurred, punishment was delivered through the immediate removal of this positive reinforcer. For both children, this condition produced a convincing drop in the frequency of stuttering. After several sessions of this condition, the baseline condition was reinstated by withdrawing the punishment contingency for several sessions. For both children, stuttering remained at the low rate it had attained during punishment. Furthermore, the reduction of stuttering was also observed to generalize to each child's conversations with a stranger outside of the clinic room, and to each child's conversations with his mother at home. These changes were also observed to be maintained at the time of a one-year follow-up.

One might be bothered by the observation that stuttering did not return to its baseline level when the contingencies were withdrawn. We earlier pointed out that this is the only way we know, through ABA experimental designs, that the measured behavior change was actually a function of the experimental manipulations, in this case the combination of reinforcement and punishment. On the other hand, as clinicians we're pleased to find a treatment procedure that produces such powerful and lasting effects. It is my opinion that the reason Martin et al.'s subjects did not show a return of their stuttering frequency to baseline rates was because the treatment condition was in effect for so long that it became permanently effective. Had they introduced the reversal condition in earlier sessions, perhaps utilizing an ABA design within some of the early treatment sessions as did Reed and Godden (1977), a reversal would have occurred to verify the functional relation between stuttering frequency and reinforcement-punishment contingencies.

In a similar study conducted in our lab with older subjects, this effect was demonstrated (Costello, 1975). In our timeout study, adolescent and young adult male stutterers engaged in conversation with a clinician. Each session contained ABA portions so that a session began with free conversation to establish the baseline rate of stuttering for the subject for that day. When stuttering stabilized, timeout contingencies were introduced wherein each moment of stuttering produced both the removal of clinician attention (similar to the removal of Suzibelle's attention) and the clinician's instruction to the subject to immediately stop talking for 10 seconds. Therefore, our timeout procedure consisted of the removal of clinician attention and the addition of the removal of the opportunity to talk at all (not a part of Martin et al.'s timeout contingency). In every session for all three subjects, this timeout contingency produced a reduction in stuttering. The last part of each session was reserved for the withdrawal of the punishment contingency, thus producing an ABA design within each session. In the early sessions, stuttering behavior was seen to approach baseline levels when the contingencies were withdrawn. However, in later sessions, stuttering behavior began to maintain its lowered rate, even when the contingencies were removed, thus matching the lack of reversal observed for Martin et al.'s subjects.

Reed and Godden's (1977) study was similar in design. However, their punishment procedure consisted of saying "slow down" to the subject each time a moment of stuttering occurred. For two children, a male, aged 5-10, and a female, aged 3-9, this contingency was effective in producing decreases in stuttering that generalized beyond the experimental treatment setting.

Another demonstration of the effectiveness of a combination of positive reinforcement for fluent utterances and punishment for stuttering occurs in a clinical report by Johnson, Coleman, and Rasmussen (1978). Their subject was a 6-year-old male stutterer who received treatment in which progressively longer fluent utterances were reinforced by the clinician's attention and praise. The consequence for a moment of stuttering was that the child repeat after the clinician any word that had been stuttered, and then the entire sentence or phrase that had contained that word. This is likely to have functioned as a punishment procedure. Johnson et al. report that not only did stuttering decrease substantially during the use of this treatment method, but the form of the remaining moments of stuttering also changed. At the end of the study, the infrequent moments of stuttering that still occurred were generally whole-word repetitions. No prolongations, and only a few part-word repetitions, remained. The authors also report, anecdotally, that this young child's awareness or concern about his stuttering did not appear to increase as a by-product of this very direct approach at modifying his speaking behavior.

Other well-documented demonstrations of the effectiveness of the combination of reinforcement for fluency and punishment for stuttering in the speech of stuttering children of all ages can be found in the excellent clinical reports of Ryan (e.g., 1971, 1974).

There are two summary statements I'd like to make at this point. First, based on my knowledge of the data in the literature, my own research

(Costello, 1975; Costello and Ferrer, 1976), and my own clinical experience, I am of the opinion that the most effective way to do this kind of treatment is to provide **both** reinforcement for fluent responses and feedback (punishment) for the occurrence of stuttering in the speech of young children. When punishment contingencies are included, the child does not cringe, he does not cry, he does not hate you. He simply figures out a lot faster what it is that he's supposed to do.

Second, I have been impressed by the experimental data and some of my own clinical experience regarding the speed of the effectiveness of this direct approach to stuttering with young children. Although the degree to which fluent speech was established in the children who were subjects in the above-described research and the nature and requirements of each treatment method certainly differed, it is still interesting to review the amount of time each child participated in direct treatment. The least time spent in effective treatment was Shaw and Shrum's (1972) three subjects who participated in only one hour and 20 minutes (1 hr. 20 min.) of fluency treatment. In order of increasing treatment duration, Peters' (1977) two subjects participated in 2 hr. 10 min. and 2 hr. 27 min. of treatment, respectively. Reed and Godden's (1977) two subjects required 3 hr. 20 min. and 5 hr., respectively. Martin et al.'s (1972) subjects participated in 3 hr. 20 min. and 9 hr. of timeout treatment, while Johnson et al. (1978) had their subject enrolled for 21 hours of treatment. Although the major purpose of all of this research was to study the changeability of stuttering behavior under direct treatment and develop effective treatment methods, most of these studies concentrated on **establishing** increased fluency and reduced stuttering in the clinic setting rather than producing generalized treatment effects, although some of them did the latter as well. Even so, the message here, for clinicians and researchers alike, is that fluency and stuttering in young children may be a relatively malleable set of responses. The older the client, however, the more intractable stuttering appears to become, as is exemplified by the treatment literature on adolescent and adult stutterers.

THE BASICS OF BEHAVIORAL TREATMENT OF STUTTERING

As all clinicians know, before one can begin treatment a careful assessment of the behavior of interest is demanded. Since this has been described in detail elsewhere (Costello, 1981), I shall not reiterate here beyond saying that it is important to have a clear description of the child's stuttering behavior, its frequency of occurrence in connected speech and in the tasks to be used during treatment, and to have data regarding the child's speaking rate as well. All of these (as well as other) aspects of the child's behavior are likely to change during treatment, and one must appreciate their status before treatment in order to evaluate improvement during and at the end of treatment.

After one has obtained assessment data regarding the child's talking performance, a treatment program can be designed. There are many ways to go about this, and I am not a person who advocates the use of a single, commercially or clinician-prepared treatment method for all children who stutter. The assessment data that have been gathered should give the clinician crucial information regarding the type of treatment design that might be effective for a given client. Nonetheless, all of the treatment that I do is based upon some common principles of treatment design that are applicable across a variety of distinguishable treatments. These principles are the principles of learning as applied through programmed instruction (which has also been described in detail elsewhere — e.g., Costello, 1977, 1980). A basic premise that I advocate, however, and would like to share with you, is the following. In the design of treatment for stuttering in young children, we should begin with the basics — with the most simplistic and uncomplicated kind of treatment format — and then allow the data from treatment sessions to provide guidance for the alteration of treatment variables, *only* if such alteration is demonstrated to be necessary.

If one is keeping track of the child's performance during treatment by noting correct and incorrect responses for every trial of every step of the program, it will be very clear to the clinician when the program is working well and the child's behavior is improving adequately, or when the child is failing and the program requires modification. When one collects response-by-response data online during treatment sessions (accompanied, of course, by periodic probes of the child's performance in more natural talking tasks in and outside of the clinic), clinical decision making becomes greatly simplified. One is not left in the position of making nonempirical clinical judgments about the progress of treatment. Rather than saying to oneself at the end of a session, "Well, he seemed to like that activity and I think he did pretty well, maybe I'll do that again for the next session," or, "Well, he seemed to like that activity and I think he did pretty well, maybe I'll move on to something new for the next session," the clinician can make a decision about the direction of continued treatment on the basis of data that are more objective than her "best guess" about what to do next.

When I talk about beginning with the simplest, most basic approach to the modification of the child's talking, I am referring to the principles elucidated in the literature reviewed above: arranging differential consequences for the occurrence of fluent utterances and moments of stuttering. That's about as simple as one can get, and we have some reliable clinical-experimental data that say this is an effective treatment strategy for young children who stutter. Why, then, should we make the task more difficult for ourselves and the child by attempting to do more than this, if, in fact, this would be enough to produce fluent-sounding speech that is used consistently by the child in his or her natural environment?

ELU Program

In the Appendix is a description of what I refer to as an Extended Length of Utterance (ELU) program (Costello, 1980) that is one version of the basic treatment we use with young children. This program is similar in principle to what Ryan (1974) has described as GILCU (Gradual Increase in Length and Complexity of Utterance). This treatment program is often a good starting place for applying the basics and is offered here simply as an illustration of one way to design such treatment.

As one reads down each page in the third column, labeled Response — the column that describes the behavior required of the child as the program progresses — it can be seen that the ELU program moves very gradually from short, simple fluent utterances to fluent utterances that are longer and longer, and more linguistically complex and naturalistic. For example, Step 1 requires that the child produce only a one-syllable word without stuttering. When he is able to do that (determined by his meeting the Pass Criterion specified in the fifth column of the program), he then moves to Step 2, wherein two-syllable utterances are evoked. Intermixed among the two-syllable responses of this step are (1) meaningless word strings composed of a sequence of two unrelated monosyllabic words (e.g., **house-car**), (2) bisyllabic words (e.g., **mother**), and (3) two-syllable two-word syntactically meaningful word combinations (e.g., **red rose**). By the time we reach Step 9, for example, the nature of the required fluent response has changed so that now the child is formulating connected speech utterances in monologue for a specified length or duration (which is 10 seconds in Step 9). The program simply continues to move the child's fluent behavior in this manner, bit by bit, until the last step in the program is passed and the child is then able to speak in spontaneous conversation in the clinic with the clinician for five minutes without stuttering.

This ELU program is designed to *establish* fluent speech, which may or may not have generalized beyond the clinic setting when the program is completed. If the clinician's extraclinic measures do not indicate that the fluent speech observed in the clinic has also carried over to the child's natural environment, then of course treatment designed to promote such generalization would be next on the agenda — but that is a topic for another paper (e.g., Boberg, 1981). Young children often spontaneously generalize their newly acquired fluency to the natural environment without elaborate transfer programs and additional instruction, but this is certainly not always the case.

Column 4 of the ELU program delineates how those all-important consequences for fluent responses and moments of stuttering are applied in this program. Perusal of this column through the course of the program illustrates the use of a token system of positive reinforcers combined with social reinforcement for fluent utterances. Reinforcers are initially given for every fluent response. As the program progresses, the token system is gradually faded out and the reinforcement schedule is gradually made more intermittent, so that by the end of the program the child is no longer relying on continuous social and token reinforcers in order to be fluent.

For most of the steps of this program, stuttered responses are followed by the clinician saying "stop" to the child as soon as a moment of stuttering is recognized — even before the child has completed the attempted word. At this time the child must refrain from continuing the utterance until the next trial is initiated. Only on the last steps of the program is the delivery of this punishment contingency delayed (until the entire four- or five-minute talking response is completed). As is well known, the power of attaching consequences to behavior is strongest when those consequences immediately follow the behavior of interest. However, by the end of the establishment phase of treatment, one does not want the client to be dependent upon such feedback or upon artificial reinforcers and punishers not likely to occur in the natural environment. Hence, these are faded out gently and gradually, so that the client learns to maintain the newly acquired behavior without artificial contingencies.

The remaining sections of the ELU program provided in the Appendix are relatively self-evident. Column 2 describes the stimuli to be presented by the clinician in order to evoke the response required at each step of the program. Column 5 specifies how well the child must perform on a given step (the Pass Criterion) before it is considered mastered and the next step is presented, or how poorly the child must perform (the Fail Criterion) before the clinician determines that the given step is too difficult and designs a branch step in the treatment sequence to remediate whatever problem the child appears to be having. The last column instructs the clinician regarding how to record data describing the child's behavior at each step, so that the child's performance can be objectively described, so that the clinician can know when to move on or design a branch step, and so that the effectiveness of the program can be determined.

The ELU program can be administered to persons of all ages, and is especially useful for children. Written or picture stimuli can be presented to evoke responses at each step of the program, but it is helpful if the child can read, so that the length of utterance emitted in Steps 1 through 6 can be precisely controlled. It is permissible to administer each of these steps imitatively, however, if a child cannot read, although the transition from Step 6 to the spontaneous, self-formulated speech required in Step 7 is sometimes difficult for children whose responses have been totally imitative up to that point. Clinicians may find that the regimented nature of the ELU program is difficult for some very young children (two-and-a-half to four-and-a-half, or so), even if the treatment is presented imitatively.

When this is the case, we generally simply engage the child in spontaneous conversation during play activities and reinforce fluent utterances of the specified length as they occur naturally in the child's speech. Moments of stuttering continue to be consequated by the clinician asking the child to stop speaking momentarily or by providing verbal feedback of some kind such as saying, "Uh oh, I heard a bumpy word," or asking the child to repeat the utterance (fluently) following the clinician's model.

In our experience it has not been necessary (nor deemed helpful or appropriate) to explain to young children our treatment strategies. We simply provide reinforcers for fluent utterances and some other kind of feedback for moments of stuttering. We do not, however, explain what the child must do to earn a reinforcer (although some of our social reinforcers are comments such as, "That's really good talking!"), nor do we explain what is the matter with his or her speech when we say "Stop," or remove a token reinforcer, or ask that an utterance be repeated. Explanations tend to be confusing to young children, rather than helpful. If the proper reinforcers and punishers are selected, the contingencies function quite well on their own. We are not so much worried about alerting children to their moments of stuttering as we are concerned about providing them with information that is meaningless and confusing. Some children will quickly, or eventually, figure out the nature of their responses that produce reinforcers or punishers and will verbalize this to the clinician. I've even known children who, having been in a program where a token is removed following each moment of stuttering, give back a token each time they catch themselves stuttering! Intuitively, it seems like a good sign if a child (or any other client) consciously understands the goals of treatment and can correctly monitor his or her own behavior. However, where very young children are concerned at least, it appears that this is not a prerequisite to the success of treatment. It would be interesting to study the role of this kind of awareness as a predicter of the speed or magnitude of treatment effects. Lacking such data, however, it is our policy not to bother the children with the rationales underlying their treatment.

Another reason I encourage clinicians not to provide elaborate explanations of the tasks presented, or the nature of the response required, or the rules for earning reinforcers or punishers, is because I like to encourage clinicians to talk as little as possible during the sessions. Maybe there's something inherent in people who like to talk being attracted to a profession that helps others learn to like to talk, and speech-language pathologists as a group do seem to be big talkers (myself included!), but that can provide problems for the child who is trying to learn. In most clinical settings, available treatment time is all too short and infrequent as it is. And if a substantial part of the treatment time is used up as clinician talking time, less talking time is left for the child. In my view, fluency and stuttering are, first and foremost, motor behaviors; and motor behaviors are learned through repeated practice. One learns motor behavior by emitting a lot of it and receiving differential feedback for correct and incorrect responses. The more opportunities the child has to produce fluent responses, the more rapidly this form of talking will become automatic in his or her repertoire.

Additives

Rate Control. Now you might ask, but what if simple reinforcement of fluent utterances and punishment of moments of stuttering doesn't work, or produces a less-than-satisfactory change in the child's manner of talking? Figure 4-1 illustrates what I shall call "additives" — additions to the basics that are appropriate supplements to treatment for some stuttering children. (By the way, many researcher-clinicians would advocate incorporating one or more of these additives from the beginning of treatment

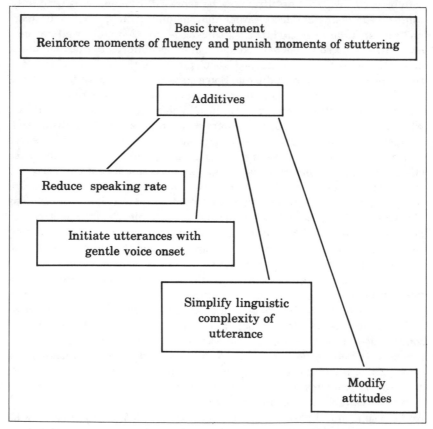

Figure 4-1. A schematic illustration of basic treatment supplemented progressively by the addition of other variables to the treatment method.

for adults who stutter because their behavior may be more difficult to change. In my opinion, too many persons writing about the treatment of stuttering in young children operate in the same fashion, designing treatment that includes some of these variations before they find out whether the simple basics are sufficient to produce meaningful changes in a child's speech.)

Probably the method of first choice is some kind of rate control, especially if the assessment and treatment data indicate that the child speaks very rapidly. To find this out, one must measure not overall speaking rate (the average number of syllables per minute when all syllables spoken, included stuttered ones, are counted), but *articulatory rate* (Costello, 1981; Perkins, 1975) (the average number of syllables produced per minute in segments of nonstuttered speech). This is the only appropriate measure of how rapidly the child is actually talking. (For a complete discussion of this issue and instructions regarding how to measure articulatory rate, see Costello, 1981.) If articulatory rate is above 180 to 200 syllables per minute, the child's speaking rate may be too fast to allow him to learn to produce fluent speech. However, there is little research on optimum speaking rates for children, stutterers or not, and so it is difficult to specify what rates are acceptable and what rates are too fast. It may turn out that stuttering children, in order to be fluent, must speak considerably more slowly than the above-proposed 180 to 200 syllables per minute, or it may turn out that speaking rate is not an important variable where the development of fluency is concerned. (It does appear, however, to be important in the treatment of adults.)

At any rate (no pun intended), if the clinician suspects that a child's speaking rate is too fast, then the basic program can be modified to require that responses not only be fluent, but be produced within certain rate limits. The best known rate control methods are those that have used delayed auditory feedback (DAF) to force speakers to slow their speaking rate through extreme prolongation of continuants and vowels, because talking in this manner allows the talker to better cope with the disruptive effects of DAF. The work of Ryan (1971, 1974) and Shames and Florance (1980) exemplifies the use of DAF and slow, prolonged speaking rates to establish fluency in the speech of stuttering children. It is my opinion, however, that it is generally unnecessary to go to such extremes to modify speaking rate in young children, and Adams (1980) points out what we have also observed — that young children don't much like DAF and have difficulty using extremely prolonged speech and maintaining it for any significant duration. Further, if one were successful in teaching a child to use this kind of speech (and it **does** produce speech that does not contain stuttering), then one would be faced with the problem of fading out this unusual pattern of speech and keeping the fluency it has generated at the same time. This has proved difficult to do with adults, and it's not clear to me that it would be any easier with children.

There are other less extreme, but effective, ways of reducing speaking rate in the speech of young children. For example, simply instructing the child to slow down and then reinforcing, at each step of the program, only those responses that are both fluent and within a prescribed speaking rate limit, has been effective in our clinic. Sometimes we model the desired speaking rate for the child, and sometimes we have them add a tiny bit of prolongation to their speech in order to slow it down and make phonetic transitions more continuous. Once again, though, any additions of this kind are more difficult to teach the child and are more difficult to get rid of later on. We have found that it is not necessary to slow down the speaking rate much below 120 syllables per minute, and then gradually let it move back up to a maximum of 180 syllables per minute. If the ELU program is being administered and the child is at, say, Step 8, where five seconds of continuous fluent talking is required, the clinician can count the number of syllables in each response the child produces. She would know that if more than 10 syllables were produced (12 five-second intervals = one minute, and 10 syllables x 12 intervals = 120 syllables per minute), the child was talking too fast. Feedback could be provided and the response scored as incorrect. As the program progressed, allowed speaking rate could be gradually increased, as long as fluency was maintained, until a comfortable conversational rate was attained. During this treatment, to be sure that altering speaking rate is necessary and is responsible for observed fluency, the clinician should allow her data to provide this information. For example, blocks of trials could be conducted where control of speaking rate was alternately required or not required. Then one could look at the data and see if slower responses contained less stuttering than faster responses.

Gentle onset. Another additive that some people use is to teach the stutterer to initiate utterances with a gentle onset of voice. I mean this to be synonomous with airflow types of treatment and treatments that discuss management of the breathstream. Adams (1980) and Adams and Runyan (1981) describe this kind of treatment with children and appear to use it regularly with certain kinds of children. Shine (1980) teaches children to whisper their responses in early steps of his treatment program, and then gradually to use louder voice while maintaining fluency until they are operating eventually at a conversational level of vocal intensity. Children whose talking style contains acute moments of articulatory closure (often described as hard contacts or silent prolongations), and whose initiation of vocalization is bombastic and frequently contains glottal stops, might be signaling the appropriateness of a treatment tactic that would smooth out those interruptions in the flow of air past the vocal folds. This kind of speech is generally initiated with a bit of breathiness which is later faded out so that normal speech is attained. Once again, getting this response variation into the child's repertoire in the first place is often a bit difficult, and getting it out again can be difficult as well, so one wouldn't want to use this additive technique unless the data clearly indicated that the basics weren't sufficient for a given child. Further, one would want to test the effectiveness of the technique (by making ABAB manipulations as described above for speaking rate alterations) to be sure that changes in fluency and stuttering were clearly due to the addition of gentle onset technique. (It has been my observation that use of gentle onset usually precipitates a decrease in speaking rate, and so it may be difficult to assess which component, slowed speaking rate or gentle initiation of voicing, is responsible for observed treatment effects.)

Linguistic simplification. Many persons conducting research these days hypothesize a language component to the stuttering child's problems. For example, Gregory and Hill (1980) state that 55 percent of 52 children they studied demonstrated problems of word retrieval (although these data have never been published for the scrutiny of others). Adams (1980) apparently believes there is a substantial subgroup of such children. He describes his treatment that requires slowed speech and gradually increasing utterance lengths as well-suited to the stuttering child with language problems, because it gives the child time to organize central language-processing functions. Among a myriad of studies investigating the role of language in the problem of stuttering are two recent articles with similar findings (Bernstein, 1981; Wall, Starkweather and Cairns, 1981). Using different methodologies with young stuttering subjects, both studies indicated that moments of stuttering were most likely to occur at clause boundaries. Since both studies were interested in the role of syntax in the stuttered speech of young children, both suggested that something about the child's ability to plan and/or process syntactic strings might be at the heart of stuttering. However, one could offer an alternative hypothesis to account for these findings. Clause boundaries often occur at the place in an utterance where the talker is motorically initiating a new utterance. Therefore, one could suggest that motor planning deficits, rather than syntax planning problems, could be related to the unusually high occurrence of moments of stuttering at these loci. In fact, in Wall, Starkweather, and Cairns (1981) and again in Wall, Starkweather, and Harris (1981), it was found that stuttering occurred most often on words that were preceded by a pause (juncture) and began with a voiced phoneme, thus providing more evidence for the thesis espoused by some that stuttering could be a phonetic transition defect (e.g., Adams, 1981; Van Riper, 1975; Wingate, 1969). Further, children appear to stutter more on longer utterances. Whether this is because such utterances are more complex linguistically, or more complex motorically, is still a question for study. The separation of language from motor issues is a delicate matter and not at all resolved in the research.

Just as I commented regarding other additives, one should not assume that language variables such as vocabulary selection, semantic relations, syntactic rules, or pragmatic functions are potential targets for manipulation in the stuttering child's treatment program unless one has data that indicate a child has deficiencies in one or more of these areas. (It is perfectly possible, as well, that a given child could have a language disorder and a stuttering disorder completely independent of one another.) For the time being, at least, my own personal evaluation of the research on language disorders among stuttering children leads me to believe that there exists no functional relationship between these two dimensions. Therefore, designing treatment with a language component additive would be low priority for my treatment (although this may be an inadvertent component of the ELU program).

Attitudes. A last look at Figure 4-1 illustrates another additive that has been considered in the treatment of children who stutter: the modification of their attitudes about communication and themselves as communicators. There are some serious questions about the role of attitudes in the precipitation and maintenance of stuttering. Even in adults, it is not clear whether adult stutterers' pessimistic attitudes negatively influence the outcome of their treatment — or even whether attitudes can be measured with validity or reliability (Guitar, 1976, 1979, 1981; Guitar and Bass, 1978; Ingham, 1979; Young, 1981). Research by Andrews and Cutler (1974) with adult stutterers showed that measures of attitude changed in a positive direction without attitudinal treatment when direct treatment for stuttering produced reductions in stuttering. There is essentially no literature that demonstrates that children who go through stuttering treatment have attitudinal problems beforehand or afterward. Turnbaugh and Guitar (1981) describe a public school treatment program that has incorporated attitudinal treatment as a significant component in the overall treatment plan. Children are first seen for long-term, nonintensive treatment directed at attitude modification, and then they are enrolled in a short-term, intensive treatment program directed (through DAF) at the modification of their speech production. Although Turnbaugh and Guitar appear to assume that the initial stage of attitude treatment is necessary for the success of the direct treatment component of their program, this was not demonstrated (or tested) by their research.

We've all noted stuttering children who were reticent about talking and who seemed to be shy or embarrassed, presumably because of the difficulty in talking their stuttering provoked. And we've all seen those same children turn into little chatterboxes as their treatment progressed and they became fluent. More significantly, though, it is my impression that most young children who stutter exhibit few signs of attitudinal problems regarding their self-confidence, their willingness to talk, and their ability to interact socially with other children or adults. Although we have no standardized and validated measures of attitudes in children yet, it's probably not helpful to engage in idle, clinical speculation, either. Until, and unless, there is some reason to suspect a crucial role for attitude in a given child, my suggestion is to stick with the basics when designing treatment.

SUMMARY

The purpose of this chapter has been twofold. One purpose was to describe the behavioral literature on the direct treatment of stuttering in young children and provide a systematic, data-based model illustrating one way a clinician could go about applying such treatment. The second goal of this treatise was to express my strong feelings that young children who stutter should be enrolled in this kind of treatment, and to prod clinicians into believing that they can and will be successful treatment providers for such children. If tomorrow you begin combing your potential caseload for stuttering children, my goal will have been met.

REFERENCES

Adams, M. The young stutterer: Diagnosis, treatment, and assessment of progress. In W. Perkins (Ed.), *Strategies in Stuttering Therapy. Seminars in Speech, Language and Hearing*, 1980, *1*, 289-300.

Adams, M. The speech production abilities of stutterers: Recent, ongoing, and future research. *Journal of Fluency Disorders*, 1981, *6*, 311-326.

Adams, M., and Runyan, C. Stuttering and fluency: Exclusive events or points on a continuum? *Journal of Fluency Disorders*, 1981, *6*, 197-218.

Ainsworth, S. *Stuttering: What It Is and What To Do About It*. Lincoln, Nebraska: Cliff Notes, Inc., 1975.

Ainsworth, S. and Fraser-Gruss, J. *If Your Child Stutters — A Guide for Parents*. Speech Foundation of America, 1981 (3rd printing).

Andrews, G., and Cutler, J. Stuttering therapy: The relation between changes in symptom level and attitudes. *Journal of Speech and Hearing Disorders*, 1974, *39*, 312-319.

Bar, A. The shaping of fluency not the modification of stuttering. *Journal of Communication Disorders*, 1971, *4*, 1-8.

Bernstein, N. Are there constraints on childhood disfluency? *Journal of Fluency Disorders*, 1981, *6*, 341-350.

Boberg, E. *Maintenance of Fluency*. New York: Elsevier, 1981.

Brutten, E., and Shoemaker, D. *The Modification of Stuttering*. Englewood Cliffs, New Jersey: Prentice-Hall, Inc., 1967.

Cooper, E. Clinician attitudes toward stuttering: A study of biogotry? A paper presented at the ASHA Convention, Washington, D.C., 1975.

Cooper, E. *Understanding Stuttering: Information for Parents*. Chicago: National Easter Seal Society for Crippled Children and Adults, 1979.

Costello, J. The establishment of fluency with timeout procedures: Three case studies. *Journal of Speech and Hearing Disorders*, 1975, *40*, 216-231.

Costello, J. Programmed instruction. *Journal of Speech and Hearing Disorders*, 1977, *43*, 3-28.

Costello, J. Clinicians and researchers: A necessary dichotomy? *Journal of the National Student Speech and Hearing Association*, 1979, *7*, 6-26.

Costello, J. Operant conditioning and the treatment of stuttering. In W. Perkins (Ed.), *Strategies in Stuttering Therapy. Seminars in Speech, Language and Hearing*, 1980, *1*, 311-327.

Costello, J. Pretreatment assessment of stuttering in young children. *Communicative Disorders: An Audio Journal for Continuing Education*. New York: Grune & Stratton, Vol. VI, December, 1981.

Costello, J., and Ferrer, J. Punishment contingencies for the reduction of incorrect responses during articulation instruction. *Journal of Communication Disorders*, 1976, *9*, 43-61.

Egolf, D., Shames, G., Johnson, P., and Kasprisin-Burrelli, A. The use of parent-child interaction patterns in therapy for young stutterers. *Journal of Speech and Hearing Disorders*, 1972, *37*, 222-232.

Few, L., and Lingwall, J. A further analysis of fluency within stuttered speech. *Journal of Speech and Hearing Research*, 1972, *15*, 356-363.

Gregory, H., and Hill, D. Stuttering therapy for children. In W. Perkins (Ed.), *Strategies in Stuttering Therapy. Seminars in Speech, Language and Hearing*, 1980, *1*, 351-364.

Guitar, B. Pretreatment factors associated with the outcome of stuttering therapy. *Journal of Speech and Hearing Research*, 1976, *19*, 590-600.

Guitar, B. A response to Ingham's critique. Letter to the Editor. *Journal of Speech and Hearing Disorders*, 1979, *44*, 400-403.

Guitar, B. A correction to "A response to Ingham's critique." Letter to the Editor re: Guitar and Bass (1978), and Ingham (1979), etc. *Journal of Speech and Hearing Disorders*, 1981, *46*, 440.

Guitar, B., and Bass, C. Stuttering therapy: The relation between attitude change and long-term outcome. *Journal of Speech and Hearing Disorders*, 1978, *43*, 392-400.

Hegde, M. Fluency and fluency disorders: Their definition, measurement and modification. *Journal of Fluency Disorders*, 1978, *3*, 51-71.

Hersen, M., and Barlow, D. *Single Case Experimental Designs*. New York: Pergamon Press, 1976.

Ingham, R. Comment on "Stuttering Therapy: The relation between attitude change and long-term outcome." Letter to the Editor. *Journal of Speech and Hearing Disorders*, 1979, *44*, 397-400.

Ingham, R., and Carroll, P. Listener judgment of differences in stutterers' nonstuttered speech during chorus- and nonchorus-reading conditions. *Journal of Speech and Hearing Research,* 1977, *20,* 293-302.

Ingham, R., and Packman, A. Perceptual assessment of normalcy of speech following stuttering therapy. *Journal of Speech and Hearing Research,* 1978, *21,* 63-73.

Johnson, G., Coleman, K., and Rasmussen, K. Multidays: Multidimensional approach for the young stutterer. *Language, Speech and Hearing Services in Schools,* 1978, *9,* 129-132.

Johnson, L. Facilitating parental involvement in therapy of the disfluent child. In W. Perkins (Ed.), *Strategies in Stuttering Therapy. Seminars in Speech, Language and Hearing,* 1980, *1,* 301-310.

Johnson, W. An open letter to the mother of a stuttering child. In W. Johnson and D. Moeller (Eds.), *Speech Handicapped School Children* (3rd ed.). New York: Harper and Row, 1967, pp. 543-554.

Kasprisin-Burrelli, A., Egolf, D., and Shames, G. A comparison of parental verbal behavior with stuttering and nonstuttering children. *Journal of Communication Disorders,* 1972, *5,* 335-346.

Martin, R., Kuhl, P., and Haroldson, S. An experimental treatment with two preschool stuttering children. *Journal of Speech and Hearing Research,* 1972, *15,* 743-752.

Metz, D., Conture, E., and Caruso, A. Voice onset time, frication, and aspiration during stutterers' fluent speech. *Journal of Speech and Hearing Research,* 1979, *22,* 649-656.

Perkins, W. Articulatory rate in the evaluation of stuttering treatments. *Journal of Speech and Hearing Disorders,* 1975, *40,* 277-278.

Peters, A. The effect of positive reinforcement on fluency: Two case studies. *Language, Speech and Hearing Services in Schools,* 1977, *8,* 15-22.

Reed, C., and Godden, A. An experimental treatment using verbal punishment with two preschool stutterers. *Journal of Fluency Disorders,* 1977, *2,* 225-233.

Ryan, B. Operant procedures applied to stuttering therapy for children. *Journal of Speech and Hearing Disorders,* 1971, *36,* 264-280.

Ryan, B. *Programmed Therapy for Stuttering in Children and Adults.* Springfield, Illinois: Charles C. Thomas, 1974.

St. Louis, K., and Lass, N. A survey of communicative disorders students' attitudes toward stuttering. *Journal of Fluency Disorders,* 1981, *6,* 49-79.

Shames, G., and Florance, C. *Stutter-free Speech: A Goal for Therapy.* Columbus, Ohio: Charles E. Merrill, 1980.

Shaw, C., and Shrum, W. The effects of response-contingent reward on the connected speech of children who stutter. *Journal of Speech and Hearing Disorders,* 1972, *37,* 75-88.

Shine, R. Direct management of the beginning stutterer. In W. Perkins (Ed.), *Strategies in Stuttering Therapy. Seminars in Speech, Language and Hearing,* 1980, *1,* 339-350.

Siegel, G. Punishment, stuttering and disfluency. *Journal of Speech and Hearing Research,* 1970, *13,* 677-714.

Starkweather, C., and Myers, M. Duration of subsegments within the intervocalic interval in stutterers and nonstutterers. *Journal of Fluency Disorders,* 1979, *4,* 205-214.

Stephen, S., and Haggard, M. Acoustic properties of masking/delayed feedback in the fluency of stutterers and controls. *Journal of Speech and Hearing Research,* 1980, *23,* 527-538.

Turnbaugh, K., and Guitar, B. Short-term intensive stuttering treatment in a public school setting. *Language, Speech and Hearing Services in Schools,* 1981, *XII,* 107-114.

Van Riper, C. The ablauf problem in stuttering. *Journal of Fluency Disorders,* 1975, *1*(1), 2-9.

Wall, M., Starkweather, C., and Cairns, H. Syntactic influences on stuttering in young child stutterers. *Journal of Fluency Disorders,* 1981, *6,* 283-298.

Wall., M., Starkweather, C., and Harris, K. The influence of voicing adjustments on the location of stuttering in the spontaneous speech of young child stutterers. *Journal of Fluency Disorders,* 1981, *6,* 299-310.

Wendahl, R., and Cole, J. Identification of stuttering during relatively fluent speech. *Journal of Speech and Hearing Research,* 1961, *4,* 281-286.

Wingate, M. Stuttering as phonetic transition defect. *Journal of Speech and Hearing Disorders,* 1969, *34,* 107-108.

Wingate, M. The fear of stuttering. *Asha,* 1971, *13,* 3-5.

Young, M. A reanalysis of "Stuttering therapy: The relation between attitude change and long-term outcome." (Guitar and Bass, 1978.) Letter to the Editor. *Journal of Speech and Hearing Disorders,* 1981, *46,* 221-222.

Zimmerman, G. Articulatory dynamics of fluent utterances of stutterers and nonstutterers. *Journal of Speech and Hearing Research,* 1980, *23,* 95-107.

DISCUSSION

R. Ingham Group Question: Our group wanted to know what your criteria are for deciding to treat a child as a stutterer?

J. Costello: What I really base my decisions on are the analyses of the spontaneous speech samples obtained within and outside of the clinic. I look primarily at two sets of things: 1) at the topographies of the behavior that I count as stuttering (and I go very much by Wingate's 1964 and Adams' 1977 articles describing kernel characteristics and accessory features), and 2) at frequency of occurrence. If a person isn't making part-word repetitions and/or silent or audible prolongations, he may not really be stuttering. We also look to see if there are things that Wingate would call "accessory features," or that others have called "secondary mannerisms," and they are counted as moments of stuttering as well. If I determine that something is a normal disfluency, I don't count it. So in my data, I have only the things that I think are stuttered disfluencies. After looking at the topographies, I look at the frequency of occurrence. If the stuttered disfluencies are somewhere around 5 percent of syllables uttered, or more, I think of the person as a stutterer. (See Costello, 1981, for a detailed description of an assessment protocol for children.)

W. Perkins Group Question: Our major question deals with a comparison of the Monterey Program, which apparently is used frequently in the schools, with your program. Also, will you address the generalization period that you include in your program which permits the child to be disfluent. The Monterey Program puts such an emphasis on completely fluent speech during the clinical period; how do you deal with the generalization period and with any disfluencies that pop up during it?

J. Costello: Do you mean the GILCU part of the Monterey Program?

W. Perkins: Yes.

J. Costello: I would say that what I'm describing as an ELU program is very similar to GILCU (graduated increase in length and complexity of utterance) in its philosophy and overall approach.

Now, in regard to your question about the within-session generalization probe: this is a 3-to-5-minute period arranged to occur within every second or third treatment session. The clinician introduces it as "taking a break," and all treatment contingencies are withdrawn (making these sessions BAB sessions in relation to time-series designs). While the clinician and child are chatting, the clinician is covertly taking data on stuttering frequency and speaking rate, so she can judge whether the improved fluency observed during treatment is beginning to show durability, at least within the treatment environment. There are people who feel very strongly that one shouldn't let the child stutter within the session. However, if the clinician doesn't obtain this kind of information, she may be misled regarding the extensiveness of the treatment effects at any given time. Therefore, I prefer to take within-session samples where stuttering is permitted in order to help determine whether generalization is beginning to take place. When you see children begin to hold on to the fluency in the session when they didn't a few sessions earlier, then you know some generalization/maintenance is occurring. It might not be showing up in your beyond-clinic measures yet, but it tells you this child is moving in the right direction.

W. Perkins: The purpose of your generalization, I think, is fairly clear. The thing we wanted you to comment on was the loss of stimulus control when the children are disfluent.

J. Costello: It's not a problem. Children learn what stimuli to respond to. When one is saying "good" and "no," those are the stimuli that have control, and the children stutter less. Further, I'm trying to be able to observe when the child's decreased stuttering comes to be under **his own** control rather than the clinician's. I'm wanting to shift stimulus control beyond the realm of the clinician-administered reinforcers and punishers. The within-session generalization probe may allow me to see if/when that process is occurring.

G. Riley Group Question: Do some children develop more frustration and fragmentation due to increased communicative stress when the clinician or the parents say "stop," or ignore the child when he stutters?

J. Costello: I have never seen it happen. I have seen a very few children in the first session be confused or mad when you tell them to "stop" or when you take away a token, but this never has lasted. Furthermore, if your program is designed well, with the steps that it should have, then they're not making very many error responses and they're not getting many punishers. If you're having to punish a lot of stuttering, then you haven't designed your program correctly. The only time the literature has shown that punishment has made somebody stutter more, is when the punishment is noncontingent, and we don't use noncontingent punishment in our treatment. The worst that can happen with the use of punishment is that your punisher isn't very effective, and it just doesn't decrease the behavior.

J. Riley: What about the involuntary block that Bill Perkins was talking about?

J. Costello: I have not seen different topographies of stuttering behaviors react differently to reinforcement or punishment. We define behaviorally everything that we would call stuttering. We don't say this is involuntary or that's voluntary. We just say the stutterer has part-word repetitions, he has eyeblinks, he has facial grimaces, etc. Whenever **any** of those behavior occurs, we do the same thing: we present the selected punishing stimulus. When they don't occur, we give the reinforcer. I can't separate things that

I think are voluntary vs. involuntary. I have never seen any evidence that they react differentially. When treatment is completed, all forms of stuttering are gone.

D. Prins Group Question: As an introduction to our group question, I would like to comment on your statement that we don't have data to demonstrate a functional relationship between what parents do as listeners and talkers and a child's fluency of speech. In one sense, we really do have very good data on that; it's the data you take in therapy which clearly illustrates that when you control the parameters of listening and responding to a disfluent child (with whatever techniques you use), you can dramatically change the fluency of his speech. That evidence is pertinent to the behavior of parents as well as clinicians, and it relates directly to our group question which concerns parental participation.

Would you comment more on how you involve parents in the program? During the sessions themselves, are they trained, and do they participate? Does this start with session one and continue through the program with both observation and/or participation? Does this vary as a function of the age of the child, the duration of the problem, the symptoms, or any other dimensions of that type?

J. Costello: We work with every parent that we can. There are, however, parents that we can't work with; for example, parents who don't come to the clinic. You know that problem. And there are legitimate reasons for that; but if they can't be there, there's nothing we can do about it. For those parents, at some point in the treatment we may work in the home and get them involved there. Usually we have parents involved from the very beginning. They observe every session. They are very good at giving us ideas for materials to use as stimuli to evoke talking. So they are actively observing and participating in our decision making. Once we develop a procedure that's working, we teach the parent how to do it. And I'm glad you asked this question, because it isn't effective to say to the parent, "Now you've seen what we're doing, just run home and try this." It doesn't work at all because people think they see what you're doing, but they don't. So we bring them into the session; we explain to them what they're supposed to do; and we watch them do it. We start by having them just count stuttering and fluent responses. Then they begin sitting in front of the child and giving the reinforcers while we take the data, until eventually they're doing the whole thing, and we know exactly that they know how to do it. I should add that a parent doesn't do a program step at home until the child has met criterion on that step in the clinic and already knows how to do it. Therefore, we don't have the parents use punishment procedures. They're powerful, and people can get carried away using them, sometimes inappropriately. We get a nice spread of benefits from these home activities. The children and the parents love it, and communication improves. The parents recognize fluent utterances that they didn't hear before, and they are pleased to achieve at home what we're working on in the clinic. Besides facilitating generalization (we assume), this helps to develop nice interactions between the parents and child, and it teaches the power of positive reinforcement that some parent's haven't understood previously.

D. Prins: Although, as clinicians, we focus on specific behavior and the consequential stimuli that change it, I believe that a lot of other "consequential" events may take place that we haven't labeled, but that may be just as crucial, or even more crucial, to behavior change.

J. Costello: I agree with you that there's a lot more going on and that's what also happens when you get the parents involved. It triggers a whole lot of nice things at home that are more than just having that parent pay attention to fluent utterances and give a token or a smile. It changes relationships between parents and children. However, the stuttering behavior of children whose parents are not involved in treatment is also successfully remediated, so it appears not to be essential to behavior change.

W. Perkins: When you get fluency ... what do children change in their speech behavior in order to become fluent? Fluency is pretty much a by-product of changes in other speaking skills, it's not a skill in itself.

J. Costello: I can't tell you. With most of the young children, we achieve fluent speech by reinforcing fluency and punishing stuttering. I don't believe their speaking or articulatory rates change. I've tried asking some of the older children: "What are you doing? Are you talking differently? Are you trying anything different?" Most of them say, "No, just trying to get the tokens." Some of them don't even know that. I'm sure accoustically there would be something different, and I would predict that it would be a little increase in syllable durations. Their fluency, however, sounds effortless and spontaneous.

I would like to add that with our type of program, people are bothered about the use of punishment and about attending to the child's speaking and not to the child as a person. The other thing that bothers people is that this type of program seems to be the kind of treatment that puts the most pressure on the child. But it doesn't seem to work that way. You don't see children getting uptight or being worried about it. They talk easily and naturally. You can see they're behaving normally; they're not squinting and making faces or saying, "This is really tough." Fluency seems to be a behavior that's very probable in their repertoire and that they can choose to use.

R. Ingham Group Question: Do you have any factors which you've identified which might predict which treatment fits which child?

J. Costello: I'd like to say yes, but I think I make that decision rather arbitrarily. I've never done any systematic research which shows that if you see this behavior, you should do this sort of treatment. I think different procedures are probably pretty interchangeable. For example, I could use time-out or extended length of utterance with the same child.

W. Perkins Group Question: We wanted to know what follow-up procedures you use to find out how this comes out and whether or not you have to use transfer and maintenance programs to get effectiveness.

J. Costello: Sometimes we have to use transfer and maintenance programs. The older the child, the more likely we are to have to do that. But I can't predict that for a given child when he or she walks into the clinic. That's why I do that within-session generalization probe: to give me a little hint ahead of time regarding whose behavior changes easily and whose doesn't. Our follow-up is governed by being a university clinic. Sometimes we do it well and sometimes we can't. Most of what I'm describing to you are clinical procedures done in our clinic, not things we have done as a part of research experiments. Every fall quarter, we have a person who is in charge of contacting every client who has been in the clinic for the last five years and talking to them on the phone. We entice them to come into the clinic, if possible. If they come in, we make a video tape, and we collect all of the data that I described earlier.

W. Perkins: What percentage of success do you have?

J. Costello: I can't tell you a number. In the last five years since we've been doing this systematically, about one-third of our clients didn't finish the program for various reasons. Some of them were doing well, and some of them weren't. I can't say anything about that group. That means that we've been able to keep track of about two-thirds of our clients who were dismissed when we thought their treatment was complete. I can only think of two whom we had to have come back, and they were both about 11 or 12 years old, not from the younger group we are talking about today. I'd say these are two children out of 30 to 40.

P. Jackson: What is the age range of the children you work with?

J. Costello: The youngest child I ever worked with was 2½, and she sounded a lot like David Prins' Case Number Two. When we saw her, she had been stuttering for 4 to 5 months and she had real genuine tension, etc., so there was no question about the need for treatment. We did a version of the time-out procedure with her. It has worked very well. We also have a little kiddoes' transfer group. When children get so they're fluent all the time in the clinic, we put them in a group together and start having them interact. It's the first time we've had enough children fluent at the same age and at the same time in the clinic to do that. They get reinforcers for the amount of talking they do in the group and for being fluent. There are no punishers for stuttering, and they don't stutter very much anyway by the time we get to transfer. They get a lot of attention and reinforcement for fluent utterances, and we teach them to recognize each other's fluent utterances and to reinforce each other.

DISCUSSION REFERENCES

Adams, M. R. A clinical strategy for differentiating the normally non fluent child and the incipient stutterer. *Journal of Fluency Disorders,* 1977, *2,* 141-148.

Wingate, M. E. A standard definition of stuttering. *Journal of Speech and Hearing Disorders,* 1964, *29,* 484-489.

Appendix 4-1:

An Extended Length of Utterance (ELU) Program.

STEP	DISCRIMINATIVE STIMULI	RESPONSE	CONSEQUENCES & ± SCHEDULES	CRITERIA	MEASUREMENT
1	minimum of 50 cards containing monosyllabic words (or pictures) within vocabulary range of client — presented without model — one card at a time. example: **car, leaf** instructions: SAY EACH WORD (added instructions regarding speaking rate as appropriate for particular clients)	fluent word/ syllable	positive social reinforcer (GOOD! RIGHT! EXCELLENT! GOOD TALKING! PERFECT SPEECH! etc.) 1:1 positive token reinforcer 1:1 (tokens exchanged for backup reinforcers throughout program as follows: 10:1, 20:1, 35:1, 50:1. The exchange rate may be altered backwards as responses get longer or when client's data indicate the need for increased motivation.)	PASS 10 consecutive fluent responses FAIL, 7 consecutive stuttered Rs or 100 trials without passing the step	+ each fluent R − each stuttered R at completion of step calculate: % correct responses # trials required to meet criterion
		stuttered word/ syllable	STOP said by clinician during or immediately following a moment of stuttering. Client must stop speaking. 1:1		
2	1) min. of 50 cards containing monosyllabic words or pictures (as above) presented in pairs	fluent two-syllable utterance	as above	as above	as above

2) list of min. of 50 two-syllable words (presented for imitative or spontaneous response, depending on client's reading skill). example: **mother, scissors**		as above		
3) list of min. of 50 two-syllable syntactic word combinations (presented for imitative or spontaneous response, as above). example: **a house, run fast, tall man**				
stimuli from each of the above three categories are intermixed and presented in random order. instructions: SAY EACH WORD, or SAY WHAT I SAY.	any moment of stuttering			
3 — same stimuli as above except **three-syllable word strings** (continually use new words), **three-syllable single words,** and three-syllable syntactic **monosyllabic word combo's.**	fluent three- syllable utterance	as above	as above	as above
	any moment of stuttering	as above	as above	as above

STEP	DISCRIMINATIVE STIMULI	RESPONSE	CONSEQUENCES & ± SCHEDULES	CRITERIA	MEASUREMENT
4	same stimuli as above except **four-syllable word strings, four-syllable single words, and four-syllable syntactic monosyllabic word combo's.**	fluent four-syllable utterance any moment of stuttering	as above as above	as above	as above
5	same as above except **five-syllable word strings and five-syllable syntactic monosyllabic word combo's ONLY** (do not include five-syllable single words).	fluent five-syllable utterance any moment of stuttering	as above as above	as above	as above
6	same as above except **six-syllable word strings and six-syllable syntactic monosyllabic word combo's ONLY.**	fluent six-syllable utterance any moment of stuttering	as above as above	as above	as above

| Prac-tice | min. 100 pictures with lots of activity in them, topic cards, objects, etc.

instructions: TELL ME ABOUT THIS (present one stimulus) AND KEEP TALKING UNTIL YOU HEAR THE WATCH STOP, LIKE THIS (click the stop watch). I'LL SHOW YOU. Describe one picture in relatively slow, simple connected speech and stop at the end of **three seconds** — stop in the middle of a sentence, if necessary and click the stop watch at the same time. Demonstrate on two or three different stimuli.

NOW IT'S YOUR TURN. KEEP TALKING UNTIL I STOP THE WATCH AND SAY OK. | continuous talking in connected speech for a duration of three seconds — (stuttering allowed)

non-connected speech, pauses, problems thinking of things to say, etc.

be sure client learns to stop as soon as the watch stops, even if utterance is not completed | positive social reinforcer 1:1

re-explain task and/or change stimulus materials

occasionally helpful to let client watch clock second hand reach the "3" | **PASS** 3 consecutive correct Rs

FAIL continue task as practice until client meets pass criterion | start timing with stop watch when client begins talking

do not initiate client's response by saying "Go!" and thereby implying a fast speaking rate is appropriate |

STEP	DISCRIMINATIVE STIMULI	RESPONSE	CONSEQUENCES & ± SCHEDULES	CRITERIA	MEASUREMENT
	(for some young clients it may be necessary to conduct this and some of the following steps as a "retell" task wherein clinician speaks for 3 sec. and then client repeats the same content in his own words for 3 sec.)	be sure client does not increase speaking rate in an attempt to complete utterance before clock stops			
7	same picture, topic card, and object stimuli as above, presented in random order. instructions: TELL ME ABOUT THIS ONE AND KEEP TALKING UNTIL YOU HEAR THE WATCH STOP, JUST LIKE YOU'VE BEEN DOING. If necessary, clinician will model each utterance until the client is able to generate utterances on his own.	fluent 3 sec. connected speech utterance (uninterrupted by clinician: monologue) any moment of stuttering	positive social reinforcer 1:1 positive token reinforcer 1:1 STOP said by clinician during or immediately following a moment of stuttering. Client must stop speaking. 1:1 (be sure you do NOT say stop at the end of FLUENT utterances when the clock has reached the 3 sec. time. Say, "good," etc.)	PASS 10 consecutive fluent responses FAIL 7 consecutive stuttered Rs or 75 trials without passing step	+ each fluent trial − each stuttered trial at completion of step calculate: % correct trials # trials required to meet criterion

8	same stimuli and instructions as above	fluent 5 sec. connected speech in monologue any moment of stuttering	as above as above	as above	as above	as above
9	same stimuli and instructions as above	fluent 10 sec. connected speech in monologue any moment of stuttering fluent or stuttered utterance over 180 spm	as above as above reminder to speak a bit more slowly 1:1	as above	as above	+ each fluent trial – each stuttered trial for every third or fourth trial count the number of syll's spoken in the 10 sec. utterance and multiply x 6 for approximate spm speaking rate. at completion of step calculate: % correct trials # trials required to meet criterion avg. spm speaking

STEP	DISCRIMINATIVE STIMULI	RESPONSE	CONSEQUENCES & ± SCHEDULES	CRITERIA	MEASUREMENT
					rate (based on all trials upon which rate data were taken)
10	same stimuli and instructions as above	fluent 20 sec. monologue	as above	as above	as above
		any moment of stuttering	as above		(for rate data, multiply 20 sec. syllable count x 3 for approximate spm/R)
		fluent or stuttered utterance over 180 spm	reminder to speak a bit more slowly 1:1		
11	same stimuli and instructions as above	fluent 30 sec. monologue	as above	as above	as above
		any moment of stuttering	STOP said by clinician during or immediately following a moment of stuttering (as above).		(for rate data, multiply 30 sec. syllable count x 2 for approximate spm/R)

for some clients it may be appropriate to increase the negative feedback for stuttered responses by adding the removal of one token for each stuttered response (response cost) – This can be done here or earlier or later on, as needed.

		utterance over 180 spm	reminder to speak slowly 1:1		
12	same stimuli and instructions as above	fluent one minute monologue	as above	as above	as above
		any moment of stuttering	as above		(for rate data count syllables for 15 sec. of each one min. utterance & multiply x 4 for approximate spm/R)
		utterance over 180 spm	as above		
13	same stimuli and instructions as above	fluent two minute monologue	as above	PASS 10 consecutive fluent utterances	as above
		any moment of stuttering	as above		(for rate data count syllables for 15 sec. of each minute of the two

STEP	DISCRIMINATIVE STIMULI	RESPONSE	CONSEQUENCES & ± SCHEDULES	CRITERIA	MEASUREMENT
		utterance over 180 spm	as above	FAIL 7 consecutive stuttered Rs or 50 trials without passing step	minute utterance, add, multiply x 2 for approximate spm/R)
14	same stimuli and instructions as above	fluent three minute monologue	as above	PASS 5 consecutive fluent utterances	as above
		any moment of stuttering	as above	FAIL	(for rate data count syllables for four different 15 sec. intervals during the 3 min. utterance & add for approximate spm/R)
		utterance over 180 spm	as above	as above	

15	same stimuli and instructions as above	fluent four minute monologue	as above	as above	as above
		any moment of stuttering	as above		
		utterance over 180 spm	as above		
16	same stimuli and instructions as above	fluent five minute monologue	as above	**PASS** 4 consecutive fluent utterances	as above
		any moment of stuttering	as above		
		more than 180 spm	as above	**FAIL** 20 trials without passing step	
17	topics introduced by clinician and client for conversational discussion	fluency (0 % SS) during two minute conversation with clinician	as above	**PASS** 10 consecutive fluent conver's	+ each fluent conver.
					− each stuttered conv.

STEP	DISCRIMINATIVE STIMULI	RESPONSE	CONSEQUENCES & ± SCHEDULES	CRITERIA	MEASUREMENT
	clinician's questions, interruptions, overlapping utterances, topic changes, etc., i.e., mirroring natural conversational interactions (clinician keeps her utterances as short as possible)	any moment of stuttering utterances over 180 spm	as above as above	FAIL, 7 consecutive stuttered trials or 50 trials without passing step	count syllables in 15 sec. interval of uninterrupted client talking, one time per two minute utterance — multiply x 4 for approximate spm/R at completion of step calculate: % correct trials # trials required to meet criterion avg. spm speaking rate for step
18	stimuli as above	fluency (0 % SS) during three min. conversation with clinician any moment of stuttering	positive social reinforcer 1:1 positive token reinforcer 2:1 as above	as above	as above

	stimuli	response	consequation	criterion	notes
19	stimuli as above	utterances over **200 spm** (unless permanent target for client will be less than this)	as above		as above
	instructions regarding new rate contingency	fluency (0 % SS) during four min. conversation with clinician	positive social reinforcer 1:1 positive token reinforcer 3:1	**PASS** 7 consecutive fluent conver's	(for speaking rate count syllables in four different 15 sec. intervals uninterrupted by clinician talking and add for approximate spm/R)
		any moment of stuttering	report to client at end of trial – do not stop client at moment of stuttering	**FAIL** 30 trials without passing step	
		utterance over **200 spm** (unless permanent target will be less than this)	report to client at end of trial and count as incorrect trial		

STEP	DISCRIMINATIVE STIMULI	RESPONSE	CONSEQUENCES & ± SCHEDULES	CRITERIA	MEASUREMENT
20	stimuli as above	fluency (0 % SS) during five min. conversation with clinician	positive social reinforcer 1:1	PASS 6 consecutive fluent conver's	as above
		any moment of stuttering	report to client at end of trial and count as incorrect trial	FAIL 25 trials without passing step	
		utterance over 200 spm (unless permanent target will be less than this)	report to client at end of trial and count as incorrect trial		

MEASURE FOR EXTRACLINIC GENERALIZATION

BEGIN TRANSFER PROGRAM, IF NECESSARY (usually will be).

5

Spontaneous Remission of Stuttering: When Will the Emperor Realize He Has No Clothes On?

Roger J. Ingham
Cumberland College of Health Sciences
Sydney, Australia

INTRODUCTION

From all accounts, the 1956 ASHA Convention in Chicago was immortalized by one of the more amusing events in the history of this profession: a fully garbed American Indian interrupted Wendell Johnson in the middle of a formal address and asked him "Are you the D-D-Doctor Johnson who says Indians don't st-st-st-stutter?" (Paden, 1970). Of course, the instant comedy was generated by the delightful juxtaposition of a famous all-encompassing theory of stuttering faced with a single troublesome piece of data. But there have also been some equally, though less colorful, juxtapositions of theory and data in recent times. There are the servosystem or delayed feedback theorists faced with those bothersome initial-word stutterings that can hardly have been the recipients of disruptive feedback. More recently, we have some ardent vocal tract dynamicists faced with the problem of explaining away the laryngectomized stutterer – perhaps we can also add stuttering during singing to their problems. In each case, there is an intriguing event, the data appear to get in the way of theory. I could list many more not-so-vivid clashes between data and theory in stuttering which probably says something about this profession's approach to this disorder. For I cannot think of another disorder that appears to have manufactured so many theories and so many unshakable devotees of these theories. The difficulty is not that these favored views seem to linger on in a dataless or data-denying state, but that their strength is such that when challenging evidence exists, it's not even recognized. The story surrounding the "recovery-from-stuttering" literature, particularly the part concerning "spontaneous remission of stuttering," provides what I believe is a fascinating example of the manner in which a committed position has exerted its influence on data. In what follows, I will recount that research, overview and synthesize its findings, and consider its unwarranted influence on stuttering.

The very term "spontaneous remission" incorporates assumptions and connotations. It generally refers to the disappearance of a problem behavior without the assistance of formal treatment. When it is used in the context of a disability, it also has a medically-oriented connotation. It usually describes the lessening in some condition or the abatement of the symptoms of a disease without any apparent cause. In some respects it is almost an antideterministic label: it carries the connotation of a mystical intervention. Perhaps clinical researchers have not intended the term to have this connotation, but the manner of its use, particularly over the past few decades, suggests otherwise. And in many respects this connotation has been influential in studies on stuttering.

Spontaneous remission in the stuttering literature is usually a shorthand description for the permanent cessation of this problem without the intervention of formally managed speech therapy (e.g., Andrews and Harris, 1964, p. 33). The research used to buttress this notion is usually described as providing an account of the natural history of the disorder. In other words, unassisted or spontaneous recovery is presumably a natural and expected event. Recently, however, many of these research findings have been subjected to scrutiny and reappraisal by writers such as Young (1975), Wingate (1976), Cooper (1979) and myself (Ingham [1976]). To a large extent these reappraisals can be simply described as searches for causal explanations for the duration and cessation of stuttering that may have relevance for treatment. They have been prompted in no small way by the quite remarkable indifference that interpreters of the spontaneous recovery research have shown to the incidence of informal, even formal, therapy activities in these studies. These are principally activities that have been carried out by parents of stutterers, or the stutterers, and which are potential explanations for some portion of the recovery process. To say the least, it is surprising that until recently, virtually no account of this literature considered this a relevant variable — a situation which seems to be attributable to the overpowering influence of Johnson's Diagnosogenic Theory.

Our knowledge about the rate of spontaneous recovery[1] from stuttering is derived from either longitudinal or cross-sectional studies. The longitudinal studies involve regular assessments over time of a population of stutterers, in order to identify changes in their disorder. The cross-sectional method surveys, at one time, a population of stutterers, and/or those who claim to have recovered from stuttering, in order to identify factors associated with either recovery or nonrecovery. As a result of both types of studies, it has been frequently argued that approximately 80 percent of stutterers will spontaneously lose their problem by early adulthood. The significance of this belief is immense. It has largely supported the view that most children who stutter will "grow out of" the problem and if they are treated, this natural recovery process could be impeded. Of course, it has also implied that any evaluation of a stuttering treatment with children, especially longterm-outcome assessment, is likely to be confounded by this high recovery rate.

GENERAL METHODOLOGICAL ISSUES
IN RECOVERY STUDIES

There are now quite a few studies that have been concerned with assessing the rate of spontaneous recovery among stutterers. They have produced a variety of recovery rates. One explanation for this variety is that it reflects the age of the population in these studies. For instance, Bloodstein (1981) reviewed some of these studies and concluded that stuttering will "disappear of its own accord" for between 36 percent and 79 percent of stutterers, depending on the age group on which the study was conducted: the wider the age range, the higher the percentage. But this rather cursory explanation invites many questions, most of which relate to the methodology used in these studies.

Rather obvious methodological weaknesses abound in almost all of the recovery studies. For example, the reliable identification of stutterers within the cross-sectional and longitudinal studies would appear to be a straightforward task, yet no study has reported that its subjects were tape-recorded or that the subjects' "diagnoses" were made by independent assessors. The cross-sectional studies have mainly relied on the subject's responses to a questionnaire with only infrequent attempts at cross-validation. These questionnaires have sought relatively general information on the role of speech therapy in recovery, and have rarely provided information on the content or duration of that therapy. Of course, this leaves ample room to speculate about what type of therapy might have contributed

---

[1]For this chapter, the term "spontaneous recovery" will be used in preference to "spontaneous remission" because the former term is used in most research studies.

to the presence or absence of recovery. These are some of the more promi-nent methodological problems that should be noted as we survey the available research on recovery.

REVIEW OF RECOVERY RATES

Recovery in Below-Nine-Year-Olds

One of the limitations about the cross-sectional and longitudinal studies on recovery from stuttering is that they have been mainly directed at the below-adult age group of stutterers. Arguably, this fact alone may have increased the probability that recovery is regarded as a characteristic of younger, rather than older, age subjects. Nevertheless, when some studies have ascertained the number of former or active stutterers in a population, then the age factor becomes evident. For instance, Johnson reported on a series of surveys (Johnson, 1955; Johnson and Associates, 1959) which identified children under eight years of age who were "allegedly stutter-ing." In the first study (Study I), 46 children, with a median age of 4 years 2 months at the beginning of the study, were intermittently observed over approximately 2½ years. At the end of that time, 72 percent were consid-ered to have recovered (i.e., they were rated as either "nearly normal," "indefinite," or "normal"). In the subsequent studies (II and III), 118 of 150 "allegedly stuttering" children (ages 2½ to 7 years) were assessed 2½ years after initial interview. Yet only 36 percent of these children were found to have "no problem" according to their parents' judgments. Why such a huge disparity?

One plausible answer appears within Studies II and III. It was reported that 50 children were assessed separately by the interviewers, and they judged 46 to have "normal speech," yet only 17 of these children were given the same assessment by their mothers! So whose data should be used to assess whether subjects have "recovered?" If the parents' judgments are given priority (as they are in some studies), then perhaps Johnson's data on the 7½-year-olds should be regarded as showing about a 36 percent rate of recovery. This also turns out to be a more plausible figure if an 80 percent recovery rate is expected among adult subjects. This low recovery rate among children also seems to be corroborated in a cross-sectional study by Bryne (1931). In an evaluation of 315 stutterers who (in the main) had attended a speech therapy clinic during their first three school grades, she found that 32 percent had recovered when they were assessed up to 12 years later. However, the role of therapy (such as it was) in this study raises some problems: it could be interpreted as retarding the recovery rate; it could also imply that even with therapy, the recovery rate in chil-dren will be not much greater than 32 percent.

The age factor is also partly evident in studies that have consulted stutterers' parents for evidence regarding recovery. Glasner and Rosenthal (1957) surveyed the parents of children "approaching the first grade level," and found 153 parents who said their child had "stuttered at some time." They reported that 54 percent of the identified children had stopped stuttering and the others were either still stuttering or only stuttered occasionally. Dickson (1971) surveyed the parents of an older age group of children (approximately nine years) and found 364 who said their child had either ceased or continued stuttering. It was reported that 53.8 percent were recovered. Intriguingly, Dickson's survey also revealed that approximately 38 percent of these children had recovered by six years of age — remarkably similar to the 36 percent identified by parents in Johnson's Studies II and III.

In short, the findings from both the cross-sectional and longitudinal studies on younger children tend to suggest that approximately 40 percent to 50 percent of children described as stutterers will recover by between six and nine years of age.

Recovery in Below-12-Year-Olds

Any endeavor to estimate the rate of recovery among children over the age of nine must also allow for the number of children who might begin stuttering at this time. This factor would tend to depress the recovery rate when it is compared with that found in younger children. However, after a fairly detailed survey of the available evidence on the development of stuttering, Young (1975) concluded that there are "essentially no new cases of any significant number after the age of nine" (p. 51). Consequently, an analysis which anticipates identifying an age factor within the spontaneous recovery process should produce some evidence of this effect across the age groups "below-nine years," "below-12 years," and "below-adulthood." Such a step-wise analysis should show a systematic increase in the recovery rates and end with close to the alleged 80 percent recovery rate in adulthood.

The below-12-years group may contain a higher reported recovery rate than that reported in the below-nine-years group. But the evidence is certainly not decisive. Milisen and Johnson (1936) reported on a questionnaire survey of 132 subjects as well as their parents, relatives, neighbors, and school teachers. They provided data on 56 stutterers, aged three to 22 years, and 32 former stutterers (ages not specified). However, they also reported that these subjects were drawn from 201 stutterers and former stutterers, and that 42 percent of these were in the latter group. (They were reported to have an age range of five to 20 years!) This is a difficult study to review because of some inconsistencies in the reported data. Nevertheless, their findings suggest that the recovery rate in the below-nine-years group was not increased by adding the higher age group. This is confirmed in another study by Milisen (1936), which involved a survey of 741 children (aged six to 18 years) who were either stutterers or former stutterers. He found that 31 percent were former stutterers, and 99 percent of this group reported their recovery occurred by 14 years of age.

By contrast, Andrews and Harris (1964) provided data from a longitudinal study which claimed to have involved at least annual assessment of 43 stutterers from birth to 16 years. They reported that 34 subjects, or 79 percent of this group, had recovered by their twelfth year. However, as this writer has noted (Ingham, 1976), not all of the recovered stutterers were followed beyond their seventh year, and a portion may not have been judged as "stutterers." In other words, there is ample reason to suspect that this high recovery rate may be exaggerated.

The only other study that provides a clue to the recovery rate in the below-12-years group is the previously mentioned study by Dickson (1971). The findings, based on parent assessment, suggested a rate of around 54 percent among children aged nine years. This is probably the most reliable figure in the light of other studies, and the increased rate of recovery which is reported to occur from adolescence onwards. This figure also resembles the recovery rate that Wingate (1976) derived from his review of relevant studies on this age group.

Recovery in Below-Adult-Age Subjects

Quite surprisingly, the recovery rate in this age group is also not substantially higher than the below-12-years group. The cut-off point for studies on this population is difficult to establish because most describe their subjects as "senior high school" students or "freshmen." So their true age can only be estimated. This problem is evident in a study by Cooper (1972), which involved a survey of 5,054 "junior and senior high school" students, in order to identify "active" and recovered stutterers.

Cooper's study was a replication of a series of survey-type studies on an older age group by Sheehan and Martyn (1966; 1970) and Martyn and Sheehan (1968). Cooper's very substantial survey identified 119 active stutterers and 68 who claimed to have recovered from stuttering. This means that only 36 percent of their group had recovered, although this was composed of a 44 percent recovery rate in the senior high school group and a 30 percent rate in the junior high school group. Nevertheless, these figures are in stark contrast to the 79 percent recovery rate among 16-year-olds suggested by data from Andrews and Harris (1964). At the very least, it implies that there must have been very significant differences between the populations used in these studies.

If Cooper's finding is reliable, then it follows that the rate of recovery from childhood to adolescence does not change very much at all. Some apparent support for this is provided in a study by Fritzell (1976) on 91 children who stuttered when assessed at ages seven to nine years. These children were followed for 10 years, and during that time all received some form of therapy — although Fritzell claimed that it was not particularly influential therapy. Nevertheless, by the time these children reached the end of the study, only 46.7 percent did not stutter. Once again, this may suggest that their allegedly ineffective therapy actually impeded the recovery rate, although this cannot be established with any confidence in the absence of an appropriate control group.

Recovery in Adult Subjects

In view of the foregoing, we should expect quite a dramatic increase in the recovery rate among adults and some evidence does fulfill this expectation. For example, Wingate (1976) has provided an account of a study by Patricia Johnson on 23 former stutterers. She found that more than 50 percent of her subjects (aged 17 to 31 years) reported their age of recovery as 15 years or older. In a similar study on 50 recovered stutterers (aged 17 to 54 years), Wingate (1964) reported that 54 percent of his subjects recovered after they were 17 years of age. Also, Shearer and Williams (1965) reported that 31 percent of their 58 "ex-stutterers" (17-21 years) recovered by 15 to 17 years of age. However, any reliance on these "recovery rates" must recognize that most of these subjects had received treatment. Nevertheless, the findings do suggest that recovery, by whatever means, will be increasingly frequent when late adolescent and adult age groups are considered.

The most complete survey on an older age group was conducted by Sheehan and Martyn. It was reported in three principal studies (Sheehan and Martyn, 1966; 1970; Martyn and Sheehan, 1968) which involved 116 recovered stutterers and 31 active stutterers who were identified from a survey of 5,138 California university students. This produced a 78.9 percent recovery rate. The findings were based on an oral reading and the "recovered stutterer's" response to questions which determined whether s/he knew the "inside of stuttering." This required the subjects to describe their stuttering and its accompanying features. Subjects also answered a questionnaire on the history of their problem. The findings suggested (see Sheehan, 1979) that 52 percent of subjects recovered from 15 years of age onward. In fact, about 26 percent reported they had recovered after 19 years of age.

Sheehan and Martyn's reports are perhaps the most significant and provocative with respect to spontaneous recovery. Among many findings, they suggested that most recovered stutterers regarded themselves as having been "mild" stutterers, and their recovery was not associated with attendance in public school therapy. They also reached a number of other conclusions from their findings, which will be considered shortly. But the finding regarding therapy is of most interest, especially when related to an almost identical study by Cooper, Parris, and Wells (1974).

Cooper et al. (1974) assessed the incidence of speech problems, and self-reported recovery from these problems, among 7,090 University of Alabama students. It is possible that these students were, on average, four or five years younger than Sheehan and Martyn's subjects (see Sheehan, 1979, p. 198). Nevertheless, the stutterers and ex-stutterers were given virtually the same assessment procedure as that used by Sheehan and Martyn. It was reported by Cooper et al. that 81 percent had recovered (compared with 79 percent in Sheehan and Martyn's studies), but when the subjects who received therapy are excluded from this group, then the percentage drops to 52 percent. Unfortunately, it is not clear from their study whether the subjects actually attributed their recovery to therapy – especially since this was not reported to be the case in Sheehan and Martyn's study.

Probably a similar-aged population was used in a cross-sectional study by Porfert and Rosenfield (1978). They questioned 2,107 students at the University of Massachusetts on "whether they were or had been stutterers," and found that 61.7 percent of the 115 positive respondents claimed to have recovered. Unhappily, no information was collected on the respondent's therapy history, or their view as to why they had recovered.

At least for the sake of completeness, it should be added that recovery may occur among much older age subjects. Shames and Beams (1956) sent questionnaires to clergymen in an endeavor to estimate how many stutterers were among their parishioners. They found a substantially smaller percentage of stutterers among the older age (above 50 years) groups of this second-hand-reported population. However, the relatively small numbers of stutterers that this method identified (64 or 0.57 percent of the population) highlights the need for a more extensive survey of this age group.

Longitudinal Studies on Recovery

The obvious problem in most of the reported studies is that they rely on recall data – be it by subjects, parents, or relatives. This should not be an issue in longitudinal studies. But unhappily, it emerges that the two principal longitudinal studies contain some problems which make it difficult to have any more confidence in their findings, especially with respect to spontaneous recovery.

The Andrews and Harris (1964) study claimed to have followed 43 stutterers from the onset of their problem until they reached the age of 16 years. Unfortunately, not all subjects were followed throughout this period and the study was characterized by a monumental 33.2 percent loss in the population from which subjects were drawn. In reviewing this study, this author (Ingham, 1976) noted that 16 of their subjects were described as "transient nonfluents" (not "stutterers"), and all were not followed beyond the seventh year. Moreover the 18 stutterers, who were described as "spontaneous remitters," were not followed after the 12th year. More importantly, on enquiry it was found that at least eight of the spontaneous remitters were independently reported (Morley, 1972) to have received "at least one form of therapy endeavor." The failure to include this information raises serious questions about Andrews and Harris' claim that "in none of these children could it be claimed that the remission was induced by treatment" (1964, p. 33). This is especially significant since no information was given on the temporal relationship between these "treatments" and remission, nor was evidence included (to be mentioned) that some of these treatments actually did reduce stuttering in these children.

The second longitudinal study was reported by Fritzell (1976). Ninety-one stutterers (identified at seven to nine years of age) were followed for 10 years in this study and almost 47 percent were reported recovered. However, these findings are hopelessly confounded by the fact that all subjects were enrolled in therapy programs throughout this period. Fritzell regarded their therapy as relatively ineffectual, but the absence of a control group means that the 46.7 percent who recovered may simply reflect the rate of therapy success.

CONCLUSIONS FROM REVIEW
OF RECOVERY RATES

What can be deduced from the foregoing? Perhaps very little more than a range of interesting issues which qualify whatever findings that emerge. But on the basis of this relatively brief review, it becomes clear that the putative unassisted recovery rate from childhood to adolescence is likely to range between approximately 30 percent and 50 percent. It is almost certainly not as high as the generally accepted figure of 80 percent. Thereafter, it may rise considerably but the reasons for this rise need to be looked at a little more closely. These reasons may also be very important to recovery in childhood and raise further questions about the nonspecific nature of the term "spontaneous recovery."

"TREATMENT" VARIABLES
IN RECOVERY STUDIES

As mentioned earlier, the role of therapy in recovery studies, whether self- or clinician-managed, appears to have received only cursory consideration. Obviously, the very notion of "spontaneous remission" becomes meaningless if recovery is associated with treatment, regardless of who directs it. It may be possible to control for therapy effects if the time of its introduction and, perhaps, its content are known. But this is difficult (if not impossible) to know in retrospect, particularly if the therapy is self-managed, intermittently administered, and vaguely reported. And by unfortunate coincidence, it is just this set of circumstances that intrudes, either directly or indirectly, into most recovery studies. Of course, this type of evidence also has dubious value if it is imprecisely reported. For this reason, while these therapy-related activities are interesting to probe, this can achieve little more than to alert us to their potential importance in any consideration of "spontaneous recovery" findings.

Wingate's (1976) review of the literature on recovery from stuttering has contributed a very different perspective on its findings. His review found ample reason to question the much-accepted notion that if a child's stuttering is either highlighted or "treated," then it will be exacerbated. In particular, he claimed there was little evidence that "unfavorable critical evaluation" of stuttering by parents of stutterers results in a worsening of their problem. Indeed, the weight of evidence may actually suggest that the methods that parents and stutterers have used to prevent stuttering have been quite successful and could have contributed much to the recovery rate in childhood. A brief overview and appraisal of the evidence which has contributed to this reassessment of the recovery studies will now be considered.

Parent Intervention
It flies in the face of almost everything we know about human behavior to accept that parents of a child displaying stuttering problems would not endeavor to "do something." Yet, that is precisely the implication to be drawn from those studies which have ignored (usually by default) the contribution of parent behavior to the high rate of recovery from stuttering among their children. It is also inconceivable that a good portion of older-aged — even younger-aged — stutterers would not seek helpful techniques (readily described in the literature on the disorder), or not use advice offered by others to alleviate their disorder. Yet, once again, that is what is implied by studies which have not at least offered a caution about the possible role of this variable on recovery — particularly among adults.

The relevance of parent intervention in recovery from stuttering cannot be considered in ignorance of certain procedures which have been found effective in reducing stuttering within a clinic or research setting. Some of these studies have been described, so it should be sufficient to recall that when some stuttering children have been briefly (but consistently) stopped from speaking, or asked to "slow down" immediately after stuttering (see Martin, Kuhl, and Haroldson, 1972; Reed and Godden, 1977), it has reduced or removed stuttering behavior both within and beyond the clinic setting. There are also other procedures which draw attention to, or alter, the subject's manner of speaking, which have been claimed to be effective in reducing stuttering in children (see Egolf, Shames, Johnson, and Kasprisin-Burrelli, 1972; Greenberg, 1970). Suffice to say, at this point, that if these procedures are used by parents or children, then it is difficult to discount their therapeutic possibilities — even allowing for the uncontrolled, or even inconsistent, manner in which parents might use them. For although these procedures may not be effective when employed inconsistently, there is, as yet, absolutely no evidence to indicate that when they **are** used haphazardly they are necessarily less effective. At the same time, there is also no evidence that these procedures are necessarily effective in reducing stuttering in all children. All that we have to look to is some evidence that they may be effective with some children who stutter. This should be borne in mind as we review, once again, some of the recovery studies. However, on this occasion, attention will be directed towards parent behavior.

In the Johnson and Associates (1959) study on 150 stuttering children, it was reported that around 36 percent of the subjects' parents, confidently described 118 of them as having "no problem" 2½ years after an initial diagnosis, and 52 percent showed some improvement. Yet, during this 2½-year period it was reported that:

> ... two-thirds of the fathers and three-fourths of the mothers indicated that something had been said to the child about what was referred to as his suttering, and of these about three-fourths reported that something had been said either immediately or soon — that is, within one month. ... These persons had made a great variety of comments to the child ... the most common of which were suggestions that he slow down, take it easy, and stop and start over. Such comments or suggestions were said to have been made as often as from five times a day to 25 times a month in roughly one-third of the cases in the experimental group (p. 149).

In effect these children lived in an environment which fairly bristled with intervention methods that could have contributed substantially towards their recovery. Yet, under these "undesirable" conditions, only 11.8 percent of the children were unchanged or worsened according to their parents. However, when parents were asked to give reasons for their child's recovery, most attributed the change to the child's growth, maturity, and confidence, or because they either allowed their child to talk more, offered less criticism, or ignored their stuttering. About 30 percent of parents could not provide a reason for the improvement.

A related finding occurs in a study by Glasner and Rosenthal (1957) which found a 54.6 percent recovery rate among five-to-six-year-olds (as reported by their parents). In this group, about 58 percent received "active correction." The parents

> ... told him to speak more slowly and to take his time; made him repeat; made him stop and start over; said the word for him; reminded him not to stutter; told him to speak more softly; got angry; corrected him; emphasized the sound of proper speech, etc. (p. 291)....

About 40 percent of parents reacted minimally, that is, by virtually ignoring their child's disorder. These data must also be related to the finding that the parents mainly responded actively when more than one type of disfluency pattern (i.e., repetitions, hesitations, prolongations, or combinations) was evident in their child's speech. But it is noteworthy that out of approximately 30 percent of subjects who were reported to be "still stuttering," about 80 percent also received "active correction" from their parents. Consequently, these "active" procedures cannot be easily related to an increased rate of recovery.

Dickson (1971) also compared the method of "active correction" used by parents with children (around nine years of age) who failed to recover and those who had recovered. It was reported that "admonishments" were used by 65 percent of parents in the recovery group and 84 percent of the nonrecovered group. "Slow down" and "take a breath" were used equally often by both groups of parents, but in the nonrecovered group the parents used "start over" and "think before you speak" more frequently. This led the author to the rather questionable conclusion that the use of "start over" and "think before you speak" may impede recovery because they interrupt rather than modify the child's speech pattern. Nevertheless, Dickson's findings show that about 71 percent of the nonrecovered stutterers were also described as "improved." In addition, 33 percent of the recovered stutterers' parents had obtained "professional advice" (it was not clear whether this included treatment), but 42 percent of the nonrecovered stutterers' parents sought the same type of assistance. Although this is not at all surprising because of the duration of the problem in the latter group.

Therapy Intervention
Some studies have endeavored to identify therapy-related activities within the background of recovered and nonrecovered adult stutterers. Sheehan and Martyn's (1966; 1970) studies, for instance, questioned subjects on their reasons for their recovery, including the extent to which they could attribute their present condition to speech therapy. When their findings

are collated (see Wingate, 1976), approximately 61 percent of the recovered group attributed their improved speech to "self-therapy," "slowing down and relaxing," or "speaking more and improved self-concept." Martyn and Sheehan (1968) also provided data which compared the nonrecovered and recovered stutterers on this variable.[1] They found that 62 percent of recovered stutterers said this was due to "self-therapy or taking some action," but this was true for only 30 percent of the nonrecovered group. The authors observed that "those who found self-therapy to be helpful seemed to approach their problem directly, by talking more, slowing down, or taking speech courses. Those who did not seemed to be running away from their problem" (Martyn and Sheehan, 1968, p. 305).

The Cooper et al. studies (Cooper, 1972; Cooper, Parris, and Wells, 1974) do not provide the reasons that subjects gave as explanations for their recovery. However, Lankford and Cooper (1974) did collect this information from the parents of the recovered stutterers in the Cooper (1972) study. They reported that 79 percent of the parents admonished their child most frequently with "'start over' closely followed ... by 'slow down.' Other suggestions frequently offered were reported to include these: 'think before you speak,' 'take your time,' 'wait a minute,' and 'stop and start over'" (Lankford and Cooper, 1974, p. 178).

Sheehan and Martyn reported that speech therapy was negatively correlated with recovery. Most of their subjects who failed to recover were reported to have received speech therapy, but those who did recover failed to indicate this as a reason for their recovery. This is perhaps the most surprising finding to have emerged from the "recovery studies," and for this reason alone it merits close examination.

The complete series of studies by Sheehan and Martyn involve 1966 and 1970 reports by Sheehan and Martyn, and a 1968 report by Martyn and Sheehan. Across the three studies, there were 116 recovered stutterers and 31 active stutterers. Yet, surprisingly, the aspect of these studies concerned with the role of therapy involves fewer than the total number of recovered stutterers, and either more or less than the total number of active stutterers. For example, the 1968 Martyn and Sheehan report involved 37 active stutterers (?), and the 1970 Sheehan and Martyn report used only 21 active stutterers. (It was claimed that their numbers were reduced as a control for severity.) But if the therapy was counterproductive, then it would be interesting to learn about the type and content of

---

[1] These data are from disproportionate samples of the recovered and nonrecovered stutterers. Forty-eight recovered stutterers were compared with 37 active stutterers, even though the ratio of recovered to active stutterers was reported to be four to one.

their treatment. Presumably, the authors also did not wish to imply that all types of therapy (including their own) are ineffectual. The only indication provided is that

> ... speech therapy as reported by the respondents, included many instances of quite brief contact, and many instances of obviously incompetent and irrelevant speech therapy, as judged by either current or the then contemporary standards. Hence caution should be exercised in condemning ... speech therapy for young stutterers from these data. For example, there were very few instances of the kind of speech therapy for stuttering outlined in the Speech Foundation of America's recent publication, *The Treatment of the Young Stutterer in the Schools.* (Sheehan and Martyn, 1966, p. 128.)...

In the light of this information, it is difficult to decide whether the active or recovered stutterer's speech therapy should be considered seriously in relation to recovery: on the one hand, it suggested that therapy was brief and irrelevant, while on the other, absolutely no information is provided on subjects who received what the authors judged to be suitable therapy. For this reason, prudence would suggest that the negative "therapy factor" in these studies has been considerably overemphasized.

The effect of therapy on the recovery rates reported in studies by Cooper and colleagues is also virtually impossible to assess. Cooper (1972) reported a nonsignificant relationship between recovery from stuttering and therapeutic intervention, when severity was held constant. But Cooper's relatively abbreviated report did not include information on the duration or content of treatment: presumably this means that "therapy" may have been little more than a brief supportive-type contact with a clinician. Indeed, there is good reason to believe (see Wingate, 1971) that much stuttering therapy during the 1960's was really supportive counseling designed to assist the subject to cope with, rather than overcome, the disorder. But this may not have been true in all of Cooper's data. Cooper, Parris, and Wells (1974) provided a very brief report on a partial replication of the Cooper (1972) study on students enrolling at the university. They found 12 active stutterers and 54 who reported that they had recovered from stuttering. Twenty of the 54 recovered stutterers reported that they had received therapy. The difficulty in deducing the efficacy of this therapy is that similar information was not provided for the active stutterers. Ironically, the only way in which the therapy's contribution can be gauged is to note that the overall recovery rate in this study (81%) is high when related to other recovery studies. Yet, this high rate is remarkably similar to that reported by Sheehan and Martyn, which, in turn, suggests the intriguing possibility that therapy may have contributed substantially to the high rate of recovery reported in Sheehan and Martyn's study.

From the preceding review, it becomes clear that when studies involving both recovered and active stutterers are considered, the contribution of "parent intervention" on recovery rates is not at all obvious. It may be that their contribution is more evident in the milder, rather than severe, stuttering children (see Glasner and Rosenthal, 1957), but it is evident that their advice is offered freely and frequently to most of the children in these studies. At the same time, among older-age stutterers there is some evidence that when subjects employed some of these suggestions they judged that they contributed significantly towards recovery. This possibility is strengthened by the findings in studies on recovered stutterers only. But before they are considered, it is important to highlight some methodological issues that emerged in the previously mentioned studies.

Some Methodological Considerations

The main weakness in the cross-sectional studies on recovery is that they hinge on the subject's ability to recall events that occurred possibly one or two decades previously. If cross-validating data or information are not provided as a control, the only method of checking the validity of their findings is via related studies. Thus, when cross-validation provides nonsupportive or contradictory data, the findings of studies which have not used this control are brought into question. Such an issue arises in connection with the Cooper et al. studies. It will be recalled that Cooper (1972) reported finding 68 self-diagnosed recovered stutterers. Subsequently, Lankford and Cooper (1974) wrote to the parents of all the recovered stutterers in Cooper's study and found that two-thirds of the subjects' parents "did not feel that their child had ever stuttered." The implication is fairly obvious: the true recovery rate might be much less than what has been suggested by this type of study. Of course, it is also equally possible that parents have a poor ability to accurately recall their child's speech quality. Although, it is rather surprising that such a high proportion of parents failed to recall such a distinctive feature in their child's development.

The reasons for differences between the parents' and the subjects' responses in Cooper's study may also be related to what they label "stuttering." In reviewing some of these studies, Young (1975) drew attention to some quite relevant findings in studies by Villarreal (1945), Voelker (1942) and Sander (1963; 1965; 1968) which indicate that "there is much more complexity than realized in assigning individuals to the categories of nonstutterer, recovered stutterer, or active stutterer" (Young, 1975, p. 57). For instance, 29 percent of nonstuttering subjects in the Villarreal and Voelker studies were "said to have been stuttering" but only about 10 percent had "called themselves a stutterer." In effect, subjects recalled behaviors that others might describe as "stuttering," even though they may not have bothered them sufficiently to warrant calling themselves a "stutterer." Similarly, Sanders found that mothers would classify some recordings of a child's speech behavior as "stuttering," yet up to a third of these women would not regard the child as a "stutterer." This difference in the basis of classification might explain the disparities among the findings of Cooper's studies. It also may explain the relatively higher recovery rates in Andrews and Harris' (1964) longitudinal study: it will be recalled that about half their recovered "stutterers" had a bout of nonfluency which lasted for less than six months. A bout of this type and duration may not have been recalled by parents or subjects as stuttering, nor indicate to either that they were stutterers.

Another bewildering measurement issue is that in many studies the so-called "recovered stutterers" were reported to be still stuttering at certain times. Recall, for instance, in the Johnson and Associates (1959) studies that 46 out of 50 children were assessed by interviewers has having "normal speech," but only 17 of the mothers agreed with that assessment. Similarly, Wingate (1964), and Shearer and Williams (1965) conducted studies on "recovered" stutterers but noted that around 50 percent of their subjects still had evident, though infrequent, stuttering behaviors. This suggests that it is possible that many of the "recovered stutterers" in these and other studies are still active stutterers but were either not detected at interview, or were judged to be normal speakers. In any event, this is a much overlooked factor which may contribute immensely to variation among the findings of recovery studies.

Therapy Effects in Studies on
Recovered Stutterers Only

Thus far, it has been argued that a relatively conservative interpretation of the evidence on the effects of parent intervention in the recovery process for children is that it is at best ambiguous. But in the case of studies using adult stutterers and recovered stutterers there is considerable evidence that "self-therapy" procedures, such as slowing down, relaxing, and talking practice, might be quite useful. This is also evident within those studies that assessed only recovered stutterers. These studies are of more than usual interest because the researcher's theoretical posture with respect to self-therapy or parent intervention is often evident and antagonistic.

One can confidently argue that during the period when many recovery studies were conducted, the prevailing belief was that the child's family environment could sustain and/or aggravate stuttering. Furthermore, parental anxiety about the child's speech, or any effort to correct the problem — especially by admonishment — could cause chronic stuttering. On the other hand, if the problem was ignored and the child's speech skills were not placed "under pressure," then stuttering was likely to disappear. Indeed, one could argue that during this time the inducement of this pattern of family behavior was actually the preferred treatment for stuttering. It follows, therefore, that if recovery does occur under these preferred conditions, it may be more appropriate to describe it as a result of a treatment rather than "spontaneous recovery." This issue is well-illustrated by Morley's (1972) consideration of the findings of the 1,000 Family Study (also described by Andrews and Harris):

> ... the part that correction of the stammer plays in its persistence is important but difficult to ascertain without constant association with the family and even with our frequent contacts it was not possible to assess entirely the part played by parent correction in the persistence of the stammer. In the children seen by us the mother was advised to ignore the hesitation in its early stages and to accept it as a phase through which many children pass during their progress towards stable speech. Again it is impossible to be certain how far this advice was actually carried out, and if so, what effect it had on the eventual achievement of fluent speech. (1972, p. 68.)...

Quite obviously, Morley inclined to the view that this counseling could be regarded as a treatment agent. But from an alternative viewpoint, there is ample evidence in the 1,000 Family Study that "correction" could have contributed much to recovery. For, as this writer observed (Ingham, 1976), the case descriptions of some of the recovered subjects reveals that they received "directives to 'speak slowly,' speech therapy, and [there was] even evidence from a mother that her child's stuttering 'stopped when corrected'" (p. 281). This type of family behavior was reported for more than half of the 14 subjects for whom case descriptions were provided. It is possible, therefore, that these correctives could have contributed much to the recovery process. However, this issue is more easily resolved if comparisons can be made between children who have been exposed to different types of environments.

A comparative study by Jameson (1955) provides perhaps the only known support for the claim that parental correction may impede recovery. She surveyed 69 children ("still under the age of 16 years") who had not attended a clinic for advice or treatment for at least a year. Evidence is provided that 70 percent of children whose parents did not offer correction were "normal or near normal" at assessment, but only 62 percent of children whose parents used correction were in this category. In the case of parents who used "persistent correction, and in a few cases actual punishment," only 10 percent were judged in the same category. But unfortunately, these data are confounded by potential therapy effects. Eighty-two percent of the children under five years of age were assessed as "normal or near normal" after treatment, and only 37 percent over five years of age reached this level. Since no other information is provided, it is possible that the noncorrective parents were mainly parents of those under five years of age. However, if it is assumed that the treated children were randomly distributed, then there is some support for the argument that correction impedes recovery. The point is even more significant when related to Jameson's claim that their treatment was virtually nondirective.

Unfortunately, it is impossible to learn whether the parents' corrective advice for stuttering had been employed beneficially or otherwise by their children. There may be some indication of the effect that it had by gleaning opinions from older-age stutterers on what they judged to be beneficial. Horowitz (1962) asked 14 nonrecovered stutterers and one recovered stutterer what they would advise to assist other stutterers: "the subjects offered up such well-worn homilies as 'Don't think about it'; 'take your time'; 'stop and start over'; 'slow down'; 'take a deep breath'; 'relax'; 'buy a tape-recorder'; and 'think that you have a right to speak as well as anybody else'" (p. 31). Similar comments have surfaced within other studies on recovered stutterers — and also at apparent odds with the researcher's theoretical position.

Shearer and Williams (1965) questioned 58 self-described recovered stutterers (ages 17 to 21 years) who claimed their improved speech was obtained without "professional assistance." There was "some remaining tendency to stutter" in all subjects, particularly those who said they recovered after 13 years of age. However, it was reported that the "factor which most of the subjects (69%) felt had helped or would help in the recovery from stuttering was speaking more slowly ..." (p. 289). Interestingly, reduced speaking rate was usually mentioned in connection with some other activity. Typical responses were:

'I tried not to speak until I was ready to slow down,' 'I began to realize the problem at that age and tried to talk slower,' 'I slowed down and tried to pronounce things more deliberately,' and 'speak more slowly and think about what you are going to say.' (1965, p. 289.)...

The relationship between these reasons and some procedures currently used in stuttering treatment is, as was mentioned, quite striking. Among the other factors that subjects reported to be of assistance were: "Thinking before speaking (43%); achieving greater self-confidence (26%); becoming more aware of the problem (22%); speaking more deliberately (20%) and relaxing (19%)" (p. 289). Against this background, it is fascinating to find that the authors concluded that their data supported treatments which use "development of adequacy and self-confidence, relaxation, and particularly with older children — greater understanding of the problem" (p. 290). Almost unbelievably, the gains possible from speech rate control procedures were literally ignored, seemingly to the benefit of more theoretically acceptable methods.

In a somewhat older group of recovered stutterers, Wingate (1964) reported generally similar findings to those reported by Shearer and Williams. Nevertheless, these studies differed in important ways. The most important was that 28 of the 50 subjects (17-54 years) in Wingate's study had received professional assistance: 22 reported that it was "beneficial," although only seven (25%) said that it was "the important factor in recovery." But, since almost half the recovered stutterers indicated that therapy was an aid, it is difficult to disentangle the contribution of treatment to the recovery rate. Wingate concluded that there were "major" and "secondary" factors that subjects said aided their recovery. The main factor appeared to be a "change in attitude." This was followed by speech practice in either varying situations or by use of control methods, changing the environment, and relaxation. (Incidentally, more subjects nominated speech practice rather than therapy as being most helpful to recovery.) Wingate (1976) observed that:

> For most of these subjects recovery was not a passive process, and there are many clear assertions of commitment and application. The obvious implication is that personal motivation was one important factor common to efforts of many of these subjects. (Wingate, 1976, p. 102-103.)...

Speech control procedures, such as speaking slowly, were certainly mentioned by some subjects, but they were not prominent reasons; although they may have been involved in the therapy procedures which were reported to aid many subjects.

In contrast to Wingate's finding is a report by Quarrington (1977) on 27 recovered stutterers who had not received professional assistance. The report revealed a high incidence of subjects who used a modified manner of speaking to aid their recovery. Twenty of these subjects attributed their recovery to either a changed attitude or a "new approach to the mechanics of speaking." But all 20 said they had made some specific change in their method of speaking. These changes were "speaking slowly," "talking more clearly," or "speaking in a deeper and firmer voice."

Conclusions on Recovery-Only Studies

When the studies on recovered stutterers are compared, it becomes clear that speech control procedures figure largely among the reasons that subjects have identified as responsible for their improved speech.[2] This factor is not always identified as the sole factor and may be closely related to a change in the subject's attitude towards his or her difficulty. This is particularly evident among adult subjects, which suggests that the high rate of "spontaneous recovery" in adult subjects is a byproduct of a self-managed (often self-designed) treatment based on a modified method of speaking. Another frequently mentioned factor in these studies was that the recovery process was usually very gradual: some of the most interesting anecdotal accounts of recovery refer to a constant and systematically managed program. In this respect, they share a great deal in common with many currently advocated therapy programs.

GENERAL CONCLUSION

The general conclusion that emerges from the so-called spontaneous recovery literature is almost inescapable — for many stutterers a program of specific speech modification, constantly managed and associated with substantial practice, probably aids recovery and is largely responsible for "spontaneous remission." The self-assisting aids that adult subjects claim to use with success are also frequently advocated by the parents of many children who stutter. These aids may well be largely responsible for recovery in adulthood, although this is less likely to be the principal reason for recovery in childhood. Presumably, the motives that older-age stutterers have for improving their speech are not found as commonly among children. That should not be surprising. But whatever the crucial factor is in childhood recovery, it is obvious that a direct attack on the problem is not necessarily deleterious.

---

[2]Shortly after this paper was read, it was drawn to my attention that it overlooked a most relevant study by Panelli, McFarlane, and Shipley (1978). They reported on 15 stutterers who were assessed initially at two to five years of age and then again at seven to 14 years. Oral reading, monologue, and spontaneous speech data were obtained by clinicians and showed that 12 of the 15 were judged to be nonstutterers at their final assessment. Thus 80 percent were judged to have "recovered spontaneously." At first glance, these data are quite persuasive, but they are limited by the small number of subjects and lack of information on whether the subjects, or others, considered their recovery to be spontaneous. In other words, no information was obtained that would exclude the involvement of "treatment factors" except that the children were not enrolled in therapy. It is also of interest that at least two of the 12 "recoveries" still regarded themselves as stutterers.

The implications of these findings are quite important for treatment. To begin with, it is apparent that treatment in childhood is not likely to exacerbate the problem, and may even be desirable. Parents should be told that drawing attention to their child's problem will not result in irreparable (or even repairable) damage. In fact, it is probably wiser for parents to be told how to manage their direct "interventions" in a much more systematic and effective manner. The evidence that "slowing down," careful articulation, and speech practice are likely to be beneficial is an important element in the management of stuttering in all age groups. It could be embodied in advice that is given to parents and recognized as a useful ingredient within treatment programs. Certainly, many of the apparently successful treatment procedures presented in this volume have employed very similar methods. Therefore, it is surely time to reject the notion that recovery may be a passive, spontaneous process. There is quite sufficient evidence available to believe that it is probably anything but spontaneous. My only concern at this point is that clinicians, like the emperor, may be forced to don yet another illusory garment by believing that recovery is **always** related to the methods mentioned above. Ideally, we will not yet again have the task of finding a way to cover his embarrassment.

REFERENCES

Andrews, G., and Harris, M. *The Syndrome of Stuttering*. London: Heinemann, 1964.

Bloodstein, O. *A Handbook on Stuttering*. Chicago: National Easter Seal Society, 1981.

Bryne, M. A follow-up study of one thousand cases of stutterers from the Minneapolis Public Schools. *Proceeding of the American Society for the Study of Disordered Speech*, 1931.

Cooper, E. Recovery from stuttering in a junior and senior high school population. *Journal of Speech and Hearing Research*, 1972, *15*, 632-638.

Cooper, E. Intervention procedures for the young stutterer. In H. H. Gregory (Ed.), *Controversies About Stuttering Therapy*. Baltimore: University Park Press, 1979.

Cooper, E., Parris, R., and Wells, M. Prevalence of and recovery from speech disorders in a group of freshmen at the University of Alabama. *Asha*, 1974, *16*, 359-360.

Dickson, S. Incipient stuttering and spontaneous remission of stuttered speech. *Journal of Communication Disorders*, 1971, *4*, 99-110.

Egolf, D., Shames, G., Johnson, P., and Kasprisin-Burelli, A. The use of parent-child interaction patterns in therapy for young stutterers. *Journal of Speech and Hearing Disorders*, 1972, *37*, 222-232.

Fritzell, B. The prognosis of stuttering in schoolchildren. A 10-year longitudinal study. In *XVIth International Congress on Logopedics and Phoniatrics, Interlaken 1974*. Basel: Karger, 1976.

Glasner, P., and Rosenthal, D. Parental diagnosis of stuttering in young children. *Journal of Speech and Hearing Disorders*, 1957, *22*, 288-295.

Greenberg, J. The effect of a metronome on the speech of young stutterers. *Behavior Therapy*, 1970, *1*, 240-244.

Horowitz, E. A follow-up study of former stutterers. *Speech Pathology and Therapy*, 1962, *5*, 25-33.

Ingham, R. "Onset, prevalence, and recovery from stuttering": A reassessment of findings from the Andrew's and Harris' study. *Journal of Speech and Hearing Disorders*, 1976, *41*, 280-281.

Jameson, A. Stammering in children. – Some factors in the prognosis. *Speech*, 1955, *19*, 60-67.

Johnson, W. A study of the onset and development of stuttering. In W. Johnson (Ed.), *Stuttering in Children and Adults*. Minneapolis: University of Minnesota Press, 1955.

Johnson, W., and Associates. *The Onset of Stuttering*. Minneapolis: University of Minnesota Press, 1959.

Lankford, S., and Cooper, E. Recovery from stuttering as viewed by parents of self-diagnosed recovered stutterers. *Journal of Communication Disorders*, 1974, *7*, 171-180.

Martin, R., Kuhl, P., and Haroldson, S. An experimental treatment with two preschool stuttering children. *Journal of Speech and Hearing Research*, 1972, *15*, 743-752.

Martyn, M., and Sheehan, J. Onset of stuttering and recovery. *Behaviour Research and Therapy*, 1968, *6*, 295-307.

Milisen, R. A comparative study of stutterers, former stutterers, changed handedness normal speakers and articulation cases. *Proceedings of the American Speech and Hearing Association*, 1936, *6*, 168-177.

Milisen, R., and Johnson, W. A comparative study of stutterers, former stutterers and normal speakers whose handedness has been changed. *Archives of Speech*, 1936, *1*, 61-86.

Morley, M. *The Development and Disorders of Speech in Childhood*. Edinburgh: Churchill Livingstone, 1972.

Paden, E. *A History of the American Speech and Hearing Association 1925-1958*. Washington: American Speech and Hearing Association, 1970.

Panelli, C., McFarlane, S., and Shipley, K. Implications of evaluating and intervening with incipient stutterers. *Journal of Fluency Disorders*, 1978, *3*, 41-50.

Porfert, A., and Rosenfield, D. Prevalence of stuttering. *Journal of Neurology, Neurosurgery and Psychiatry*, 1978, *41*, 954-956.

Quarrington, B. How do the various theories of stuttering facilitate our therapeutic approach? *Journal of Communication Disorders*, 1977, *10*, 77-83.

Reed, C., and Godden, A. An experimental treatment using verbal punishment with two preschool stutterers. *Journal of Fluency Disorders*, 1977, *2*, 225-233.

Sander, E. Frequency of syllable repetitions and "stutterer" judgments. *Journal of Speech and Hearing Disorders*, 1963, *28*, 19-30.

Sander, E. Comments on investigating listener reaction to speech disfluency. *Journal of Speech and Hearing Disorders*, 1965, *30*, 159-165.

Sander, E. Interrelations among the responses of mothers to a child's disfluencies. *Speech Monographs*, 1968, *35*, 187-195.

Shames, G., and Beams, H. Incidence of stuttering in older age groups. *Journal of Speech and Hearing Disorders*, 1956, *21*, 313-316.

Shearer, W., and Williams, J. Self-recovery from stuttering. *Journal of Speech and Hearing Disorders*, 1965, *30*, 288-290.

Sheehan, J. Current issues on stuttering and recovery. In H. Gregory (Ed.), *Controversies About Stuttering Therapy*. Baltimore: University Park Press, 1979.

Sheehan, J., and Martyn, M. Spontaneous recovery from stuttering. *Journal of Speech and Hearing Research*, 1966, *9*, 121-135.

Sheehan, J., and Martyn, M. Methodology in studies of recovery from stuttering. *Journal of Speech and Hearing Research*, 1967, *10*, 396-400.

Sheehan, J., and Martyn, M. Stuttering and its disappearance. *Journal of Speech and Hearing Research*, 1970, *13*, 279-289.

Villarreal, J. The semantic aspects of stuttering in nonstutterers: Additional data. *Quarterly Journal of Speech*, 1945, *31*, 477-479.

Voelker, C. On the semantic aspects of stuttering in nonstutterers. *Quarterly Journal of Speech*, 1942, *28*, 78-80.

Wingate, M. Recovery from stuttering. *Journal of Speech and Hearing Disorders*, 1964, *29*, 312-321.

Wingate, M. The fear of stuttering. *Asha*, 1971, *13*, 3-5.

Wingate, M. *Stuttering: Theory and Treatment*. New York: Irvington, 1976.

Young, M. Onset, prevalence, and recovery from stuttering. *Journal of Speech and Hearing Disorders*, 1975, *40*, 49-58.

DISCUSSION

W. Perkins Group Question: How would you design a valid and reliable recovery study that would solve the research problems you've overviewed?

R. Ingham: I really don't think that the question can be answered satisfactorily. Such a study might have to be confined to primitive societies or societies where there is no generally recognized procedure for treating stuttering. I don't think that would be an entirely impossible project to conduct if you just wanted to get some general ideas. But, even then, there may be as many reasons for recovery in that sort of society, that we may not be sensitized to measure. I think a more practical approach is to consider whether the questions that we might be concerned with in a long-term study can be answered in fairly short-term studies. For example, whether certain sorts of activities exacerbate or don't exacerbate stuttering, or whatever. I think these can be answered more easily in some form of controlled experimental environment. My concern has been that there has existed an antideterministic attitude towards "spontaneous remission" which has negated the search for many worthwhile factors that might be responsible for sustained change. And I think that the search for these factors is where the pay-off is likely to be in this type of investigation.

G. Riley Group Question: Is there a positive side to the studies that you've cited? In other words, are there assertions which can be supported by these studies and, if so, what are they?

R. Ingham: I think there are interesting similarities between some of the early research investigations on recovery from stuttering and the tobacco industry's research on smoking and lung cancer. I think they both include some committed parties who would dearly like to have found examples to support their cases; stutterers who were worsened by parent intervention and smokers who are inured against lung cancer by smoking cigarettes. The fact that parent intervention has not been shown conclusively to retard recovery from stuttering is a positive sign. Out of all the data collected thus far there is no evidence that drawing attention to stuttering, stopping the child when he stutters, or other admonishments, aggravate the problem in any way. On the other hand if we accept that stuttering is able to be controlled by environmental consequences, then it's surely conceivable that environmental factors could be arranged to reinforce stuttering or create conditions that will sustain it.

D. Prins Group Question: If there were any pattern that emerged from those cross-sectional studies, it appeared to be a sort of biomodal nature of recovery. We got a percentage of supposed self-recovery before age 9, and then nothing changed much until we got to something like age 16, 17, and above. The percentages never changed in between. If that were so, what would it mean? Are there different subjects in these groups? What might we conclude about the factors involved?

R. Ingham: Well, I'm drawn in two directions by this sort of issue. One is the "Kiddian direction"; the direction forced upon us by the influential work of Kenneth Kidd on genetics. That would lead you to suspect that there has got to be some genetic factor that is likely to be either exacerbated by the environment or sustained by it, or whatever. The other direction is that the factors retarding recovery in early childhood may be occurring in families. If we accept that certain activities in families may induce recovery, surely it is possible that there are others that might prevent it. There's precious little research that even addresses this issue, so they are only my best broad guesses.

W. Perkins Group Question: What suggestions would you make to parents, particularly regarding the kinds of publications that have suggestions such as "If Your Child Stutters" (Speech Foundation of America), Johnson's Open Letter, etc.? How would you change them, or would you rewrite them?

R. Ingham: I certainly suggest they be rewritten. That really is an interesting question because in our audience we have the forthcoming president of the American Speech Language and Hearing Association (Dr. Fred Minifie), the recent editor of *JSHD* (Dr. Perkins), and the current editor of *JSHD* (Dr. Costello); people who could surely help put together some more appropriate information. Especially needed is information for pediatricians. In my experience, they make enormously influential suggestions to parents, such as not doing anything about the problem, etc. We are overdue for some publications that tell parents, "If your child is showing certain sorts of speech behaviors, get him or her to a speech pathologist immediately." If parents were simply told that telling your child to "slow down," "take it easy," or whatever, provided it is done sensibly and sensitively, it is unlikely to harm the child; and from what we have learned here, is probably going to help the child.

Just a brief little rider to that statement. I mentioned that there's no evidence that haphazard delivery of contingencies is likely to be nontherapeutic. I think it would be very interesting to design studies where there is a schedule of response-contingent stimulation that emulates the parent behaviors we have been worried about. It may well be that these contingency schedules are effective in modifying stuttering.

G. Riley: I would like to follow up your initial point. Let's assume that we were to get the pediatricians to send these families to a speech pathologist. I suspect things in Australia are about like they are here. I'm wondering what percentage of the speech pathologists would be prepared to answer their questions? I suspect that at least 70 percent of practicing speech pathologists would say we don't want to see this child until he's 6 or 7.

R. Ingham: You are probably right. At some point somebody has got to come out and state that the weight of evidence is now such that clinicians must step in and do something. How much more information do we need before we should tell clinicians that they have a responsibility to start doing something about very young children. It may well be something that an ASHA committee could address itself to, although you and I know the sort of opposition that that would receive.

G. Riley: But another route might be to try to work it into medical education to educate medical interns. It seems to be they're still receiving 1950s information. These are the doctors who will be practicing for the next 40 years.

R. Ingham: We are beginning to do this in Australia. Some publicity has been given to this issue in medical journals in Australia, and I think that now we're seeing the consequences. We now see a much larger number of very young children who stutter.

J. Costello Group Question: Do you have any kind of guidelines that you operate with yourself, or that you teach your students, to help sort out this literature so that clinicians can be more discriminating?

R. Ingham: I suppose that there are a few guidelines that we've all started to accept as necessary, but not necessarily sufficient conditions, for evaluating research. Slowly we've gravitated towards a situation where, for example, you have been prepared to instruct your *JSHD* editorial consultants that acceptable manuscripts should contain certain sorts of information. Those sorts of minimal information that seem to be necessary for these types of studies are reliable and cross-validated data as well as concern for the general validity of the study. I think that slowly we are starting to realize that unless data are measured independently with pertinent controls for certain influential variables, then we should be very suspicious of the study. Now, I think that the situation with the recovery studies is one where all of the possibilities for nonreliable judgments, lack of cross-validation, etc., are rife. I think that the evaluative process comes down to exercising judgments based on our training as scientists. All clinicians should be scientists: they should be concerned about collecting data, evaluating the quality of those data, ensuring that assessments occur under reasonably controlled conditions, etc., etc. They are all part and parcel of clinical practice. Clinicians have developed a healthy suspicion about the long-term effects of stuttering therapy. They've developed it because of their awareness that certain sorts of clinically relevant factors have not been addressed in certain studies. They are the sorts of guides that I use. I operate on the simple principle that if these factors have not been taken into account, then you can bet that there's a high probability that this is a problem for the study.

The other important point out of all of this is that time and again interpretations of data have been made and those interpretations have stuck. I can't give you any better advice than to always go to the original study. The interpreters of these studies have made many mistakes, and I certainly wouldn't exclude myself. We just have to be very, very careful to look at the sources of interpreters' conclusions.

W. Perkins: It seemed to us that the major thrust of your objection to the recovery studies is that spontaneous recovery was being mixed in with treatment effects and parental intervention effects. And so we had two questions: what difference does it make whether they recovered with parental intervention or whether they just recovered; however, they recovered? And in terms of the estimates of recovery that come in somewhere around 75-80 percent, are they way off or are they reasonably intact?

R. Ingham: The last question first. I think the figures are reasonably intact provided you're prepared to throw in the effects of treatment and everything else. I guess that comes back to the first part of the question — what does it matter anyhow? Well, it matters to the extent that I believe that the position had been reached, even very recently, that most texts accepted that there would be a natural spontaneous recovery rate of around about 75-80 percent by mid-adolescence. I believe that was interpreted to mean that if you don't treat them, about four-fifths will recover by themselves; that also depended on parents, or whoever, not doing anything to exacerbate it. Now, if we break down that figure and look at it carefully, then about 25 percent of that 75-80 percent look like byproducts of fairly direct treatment. But even then, in many studies the so-called "recoveries" have not even recovered.

D. Prins: What you seem to be getting at, is that whether one calls it self-recovery or not, if you look closely, something is almost always done. And no matter who it's done by, the person, the parents, or the professional, what is done seems to be similar in many cases.

R. Ingham: Generally I believe that's right. I just wish they would wipe away the term "spontaneous" and talk about recovery and unidentified causes of recovery, or words to that effect. All of our principal texts continue to use the term "spontaneous recovery," quite misleadingly, I believe.

W. Perkins: Well your objection to it really is that it implies a passive posture on the part of not only the parents and the clinician but also the child. The part of it that would interest me most would be: How passive is the child? I would be interested in learning what changes occurred in the child; in terms of either reacting to changes in the environment, or changes in the way he manages his own speech, or changes for whatever reason. What changes does he make to account for the recovery?

R. Ingham: Maybe it's the sort of thing Dave was alluding to with respect to frustration. Under those circumstances, it seems entirely understandable that a person would try to work out strategies to try to control this problem. He might come up with solutions that are remarkably like our current treatments, or some that are not.

W. Perkins: Before we leave this, I think we've got to use your injunction against leaping to the opposite conclusion; to recognize that we may fall into the same trap.

R. Ingham: Exactly.

6

Issues and Perspectives

David Prins
Roger J. Ingham

The preceding chapters have offered a blend of theory and pragmatism from a group of authors with diverse academic backgrounds, clinical and laboratory experience, and opinions. In this chapter we will highlight selected issues that emerged from the presentations and discussions at the time of the conference.

ORIGINS OF DISFLUENCY AND STUTTERING

Since the 1930s, arguments about the origins of stuttering have waxed and waned in support of (1) a single 'core' physiological factor that serves to interrupt speech fluency and thereby leads to stuttering, vis-a-vis (2) many possible factors that contribute to speech fluency failures to which the child may react by producing stuttered speech. Both arguments, though not central to the theme of the conference, appear in chapters one and two. The apparent extremes of opinion are represented on the one hand by Perkins: stuttering exists only in the presence of an 'involuntary' block in speech fluency that presumably results from a single physiological variable; and on the other hand by Prins: stuttering grows from the child's reactions of frustration and tension to his own speech fragmentations which may result from many different contributing factors.

The essential difference between these points of view lies not with the observation that some sort of 'block' seems essential for the occurrence of a real stuttering instance (at least in the chronic stutterer), but rather with the explanation of the origins of that 'block.' It could result from a single, genetically determined physiological variant, and it is equally possible that it could result from a child's persistent reactions to his own speech fluency failures, reactions that ultimately trigger uncontrollable spasms involving one or more of the valving mechanisms required for normal vocalization (e.g., the larynx). Thus, even though we can find evidence in the chronic stutterer of fluency breakdowns associated with certain physiological phenomena, the history of those phenomena in relation to the essential factors that produce stuttering remains a riddle.

The solution to the riddle, however, is not only important to theorists; it is important to clinicians, as well, and that is what ties the Perkins chapter to others in this book. Some questions pertinent to treatment include:

Is regression following treatment of the **adult** stutterer such an extreme problem because of our failure to be able to reliably identify the 'block' and thereby our failure to consistently direct treatment towards that behavior?

Might the 'blocking mechanisms' be more successfully modified in treatment by the judicious use of biofeedback? ... and, more pertinent to the theme of this book. ...

Is early intervention for stuttering more successful because it intercedes before the 'blocking mechanisms' are fully established?

SPEECH DISFLUENCY CHARACTERISTICS
THAT FORM THE BASES FOR INTERVENTION

Are there characteristics of speech disfluency in the young child clearly signaling the need to intervene? Answers to this perennial question almost always involve some qualification, and rightly so, since the word 'intervention' can imply many different kinds of programs.

Direct Intervention with the Child. When combinations of certain 'abnormal' disfluencies are apparent in more than 3 percent of a child's utterances, the Rileys favor intervention. Concerning speech repetitions these include: repetitions of part words or monosyllabic words, when there are often multiple repetitions of these elements prior to success in uttering the word, and when the repetitions are characterized by a loss of articulatory/phonatory continuity. Concerning speech arrests and prolongations these include: sounds prolonged 1.5 seconds or longer and phonatory stoppages or articulatory fixations of .5 second or longer.

Among the authors and conference participants these criteria produced no dissenting points of view. Costello (see her chapter's discussion questions) speaks of a somewhat different disfluency percentage figure, but there was tacit agreement that when the characteristics of speech disfluency reviewed above are present in the daily speech pattern of a child, it signals the need for direct intervention.

Parental Intervention with Child Observation. When disfluencies are not of the type reviewed above, but are persistent and sufficient to produce concern by a referral source, a structured fluency-monitoring and parent-reporting program is recommended by the Rileys. Prins suggests that persistence of repetition disfluencies alone (i.e., multiple repetitions before completing an utterance, and the presence of disfluency in the simplest, least stressful circumstances), even when they are of polysyllabic words and phrases, can be the basis for intervening with a structured parental observation and monitoring program.

The essence of these positions is that the speech disfluency characteristics of the very young child can, and should, be used as essential signs for early intervention, and their presence should so motivate the clinician and responsible referral sources.

TECHNIQUES FOR DIRECT INTERVENTION WITH THE CHILD

There is a clear difference in emphasis between Costello and the Rileys pertaining to the initiation of treatment programming (1) to directly establish fluent speech (Costello); and (2) to build speech/language support processes (Rileys). Part of the reason for this difference may result from the different kinds of cases seen most frequently by these authors. For example, the Rileys make it evident that children referrred to their practice are often those with severe/complicated disorders who have failed to respond to more traditional approaches. On the other hand, there is considerable similarity among these authors in the recommended directness of approach. All suggest, when intervening with the young child, that clinicians define and understand behavioral objectives and carefully program activities to bring them about.

The importance of clinician reinforcement of responses is highlighted by Costello, Prins, and the Rileys. The rationale, however, is not always the same. In order to extinguish stuttering and instate fluent speech, Costello emphasizes the use of both punishment and positive reinforcement procedures to provide specific consequences, respectively, for stuttering and for fluent speech. In contrast, Prins recommends that positive reinforcement be used chiefly to secure the child's correct participation in the therapeutic activity, allowing fluent speech (that is assumed to be positively self-reinforcing) to emerge and become established. The difference of opinion and interpretation in this case may, at least in part, be attributed to the age of the children. Prins has directed his comments exclusively to preschool children (age two to four), whereas Costello, who includes that age group, also includes programs for children who are considerably older.

Involvement of Parents

The profession has for many years emphasized parental involvement when working with the young child who stutters, and pamphlets, articles, and chapters on the subject are available by the score. This literature has created the impression that parents should be counseled generally about how to, and how not to, listen, speak, discipline their children, etc. Although there is no evidence that direct harm will come from such well-intentioned advice, there is also no evidence that any good will come from it either. Furthermore, if activities with parents lack specificity and yield no data or measures of any kind, there will be no evidence to demonstrate the effects of this aspect of treatment or the importance of it to the outcome of the overall program.

The contributing authors have restated the importance of involving parents. But beyond general counseling, they emphasize the need to assure that parents are observing and doing specific things; that they are providing data upon which clinical decisions and judgments can be made. As participants in the treatment program parents should:

be taught to use protocols to structure their observations and to assure accuracy;

participate in treatment sessions and learn to record data and reinforce responses;

serve as 'clinicians' in order to transfer to the home environment changes that have been established in the clinic.

Without this kind of involvement, that portion of treatment in which parents participate will lack the precision to make it effective and the data base necessary to help the clinician, over time, to evaluate treatment and to modify and develop new strategies.

TRANSFER, GENERALIZATION, AND MAINTENANCE OF FLUENT SPEECH

Treatment programs for the older child and adult stutterer are plagued by problems associated with securing and maintaining speech fluency changes outside the clinic. According to the contributing authors, treatment for the very young child, while not free of these problems, finds them less formidable. Prins has taken the position that, what Ingham later labeled "natural generalization," happens very quickly with the preschool child, in most cases as a result of changes that occur in the communication environment at home. He believes that fluency enhancement activities with the child serve primarily to provide the simplified stimulus/response parameters that (1) allow the child's capacity to speak without stuttering to emerge, and (2) give the parents models to practice so that they can subsequently use the activities at home. Prins does not believe that he is teaching the preschool child fluent speech responses by a series of programmed sequences that will form the basis for transfer activities and subsequent generalization. In contrast, Costello presents a sequenced program to teach fluent responses that will be followed in many, if not all, cases by transfer activities. These substantial differences between Costello's and Prins' points of view regarding the essential ingredients of effective treatment will await the benefits of clinical research to determine which factors are crucial to treatment gains within their therapy formats. Setting aside such differences, however, it is clear that, among the contributors, there is strong agreement that transfer and generalization occur much more rapidly with the very young child than they do with the older child and adult.

As with transfer and generalization, maintenance of speech fluency with the young child appears to be a more likely outcome of treatment than it does when therapy for stuttering is initiated later in life. The Rileys and Costello both present evidence that helps to support this conclusion.

THE CASE FOR EARLY INTERVENTION

No issue concerning the treatment of stuttering is as tied to the disorder's folklore as the case for, or against, early intervention. The impact of Wendell Johnson's theory, as interpreted by the profession and the laity, has had an immobilizing effect. In spite of no clear cause-effect evidence to support it (and considerable evidence to negate it), the belief remains intransigent that calling attention to disfluency in a young child may "cause" a problem of stuttering to emerge. The fear that this could (will) happen has been so widely held in our own and in the medical profession, that in the face of even the clearest evidence that a child is having problems speaking fluently, our profession has, with a seemingly singular voice, given the advice to pay no attention — to ignore it. As an antidote, the contributors to this text have harmonized on a different note: **when a young child shows persistent and unusual signs of disfluent speech** (see definitions elsewhere in this and other chapters), **intervene** — directly with the child and with the parents. No other message of the conference was spoken so clearly or with such intensity. It results from evidence found in clinical successes (Costello, Prins, Rileys) and in the literature (Ingham). We believe the profession should embrace this information and thereby transmit it to the public and other professions that provide services to young children.

Index

Accessory features of stuttering, 46
Apprehension and stuttering, 9, 10-11, 16, 19
Articulatory rate, 85, 96
Assessment procedures:
  attending disorders, 48 ,50
  attitudes, 53
  auditory processing, 45, 51-52, 65
  behavioral areas, 45, 79
  oral motor coordination, 45, 50-51
  parent interview, 44-45
  sentence formulation ability, 45, 52
  speech sampling, 45
Attitudes:
  child, 53, 54, 64
  parental, 53, 64
Auditory feedback, 8, 12

Blockage of Speech:
  involuntary, 10, 11, 13-14, 16, 19-20, 94-95, 141
  mechanisms of, 13, 15, 141-142
  phonatory, 12, 19, 46, 142
  spasm, 142
  treatment implications, 142

Clinician:
  as researcher, 69-70, 138
  attitudes toward stuttering, 71
  role and definition, 69-70
Communicative pressure and stress, 6, 15, 28, 53, 94
Component model of stuttering, 48, 60, 65-66
Conditions that increase stuttering, 5
Conditions that reduce stuttering, 5
Continuity Hypothesis (Bloodstein), 22, 24, 26, 29, 36
Covert stutterers, 10

Definition of stuttering, 2, 7, 9-10
Delayed auditory feedback (DAF), 7, 12, 13-14, 15, 16, 17, 18, 19, 85
Distractibility, 50

ELU Program, 81-82, 88, 99-112

Faked stuttering, 10
Fluency monitoring program, 47
Formant transitions, 13
Fragmentation and Tension Hypothesis (Bloodstein), 22, 24, 36
Fragmentation of speech, 23-24, 25, 33, 141
Frustration: role in stuttering, 9, 10, 11, 16, 24-25, 36, 37, 39, 40, 50, 94, 141
Fundamental vocal frequency, 14, 15-16, 18

Genetic transmission of stutterng, 4, 6, 8, 137
GILCU Program, 81, 93
Glottal vibration, 18

Hyperactivity, 50

Inheritance of stuttering, 4, 11
Insecurity in stutterers, 6
Interaural feedback disparity, 15
Intervention—Basic issues:
  criteria for, 26-27, 33, 45-47, 93
  direct vs. indirect, 71-72, 73
  emergency circumstances, 34
  how to intervene, 26, 27
  intensiveness of, 27, 33-34, 37
  postponement of, 40, 43
  timing—need for early intervention, 43-44, 70-71, 89, 138, 143, 145
  with whom to intervene, 26, 27

Intervention—Levels:
    I - nonchronic stuttering, 45-47
    II - chronic stuttering—modifica-
        tion of underlying components,
        47-54, 63-64, 66
    III - chronic stuttering—modifica-
        tion of speech symptoms, 54-58,
        63-64

Laryngeal control and stuttering, 6-7,
    11-12, 13, 14, 18
Laryngectomized stutterers, 12, 113
Lipped speech, 5, 12

Monterey Program, 93
Motor speech planning, 7

Neurological components of stuttering,
    48

Origins of stuttering:
    Bloodstein, Oliver, 6
    Brutten, Eugene, 6
    environmental factors, 72
    Johnson, Wendell, 5, 71, 113, 114,
        145
    Perkins, William, 14-16, 141
    Prins, David, 24-26, 141
Outcome of treatment:
    clinical followup, 59, 97
    establishment, transfer, generaliza-
        tion, and maintenance, 35, 81, 93,
        97, 144-145
    expectancy, 26, 29, 35, 37, 41, 67
    rating scales, 59-60
    sampling procedures, 59, 97
    spontaneous (natural) generaliza-
        tion, 36, 37, 41, 81, 144
    speed of fluency achievement, 36,
        37, 41, 79
    studies of:
        effectiveness of contingent re-
            inforcement, 75
        fluency reinforcement, 73-76,
            77-78
        punishment of stuttering, 73-74,
            76-78

Perservation, 50
Phases of stuttering (Bloodstein), 3-4
Physical concomitants of stuttering, 46
Prediction of stuttering, 5
Prevalence of stuttering, 4
Prevention of chronic stuttering, 27
Publications for parents and
    professionals, 137
Punishment of disfluency, 6

Real stuttering, 10
Recovery from stuttering (spontaneous
    remission):
        contributing factors identified by
            subjects:
                attitude change, 130, 131
                relaxing, 130, 131
                slowing down, 130, 131
                speaking deliberately, 130
                self confidence, 130
                thinking before speaking, 130
        definition of, 114-115, 121
        effect of direct intervention upon,
            132, 139
        methodologic limitations of studies:
            definitions of "stuttering," 127,
                128
            identification and classification
                of stutterers, 115, 120, 127-128
            parental intervention, 121,
                122-124, 125, 128, 129, 130
            recall data, 120, 127
            researcher bias, 128
            self therapy effects, 128
            speech therapy effects, 115,
                116, 119, 120-121, 124-127,
                129, 130, 131
        misinterpretation of, 114, 133, 139
        recover rate, effects of:
            age, 115, 116, 117, 120-121
            parental intervention, 127
            speech therapy, 116, 119, 120,
                126
Reliability of stuttering judgments, 10
Relapse of stuttering, 20

Spectrographic evidence of stuttering,
    12-13
Servosystem theory, 18

Speech disfluencies:
 abnormal, 45-46
 articulatory fixations, 24, 25, 26,
  33, 142
 and language acquisition, 23, 41,
  87-88
 as signals for intervention, 27, 33,
  36, 40, 45-46, 142-143, 145
 as signs of speech improvement, 29
 classification of, 2, 45
 deep and surface aspects, 22-23,
  24, 26
 distribution of, 23
 effect *on* speech timing, 25
 normal, 3, 45, 54
 of function words, 23
 overlap of in stuttering and
  normal-speaking children, 21-22
 parental effects upon, 72, 95
 persistence of, 33, 36, 40, 143
 prolonged sounds, 2, 24, 33, 46,
  142
 reliable judgments of, 2
 sound/syllable (part-word) repetitions, 2, 9, 23, 24, 45-46
 stuttered, 3
 whole word repetitions, 23, 24, 45
Speech fear, 15
Stuttering Prediction Instrument, 45

Tension:
 as a signal for intervention, 27, 32,
  33, 34, 46
 evidence of in speech disfluency,
  25-26
 role in stuttering, 10, 11, 22, 24,
  25, 26, 36, 141
Therapy activities with parents:
 as part of environmental management; 41, 53, 72-73, 96
 attitude modification, 54, 58, 64-65
 child observation, 33-34, 39
 empirical evidence concerning
  effectiveness, 72-73, 95
 need for specificity, 39, 95, 144
 participation in child treatment
  sessions, 40, 95, 144
 self observation, 34, 39
 training in reinforcement-for-
  fluency procedures, 75-76, 95, 144
 use of punishment, 95

Therapy activities with children:
 as a model for parents, 35
 air flow management, 57, 86
 attending, 64
 auditory processing program, 52
 behavioral modification techniques:
  behavioral assessment, 79-80
  differential consequences, 80,
   143
  generalization probe, 80, 93, 97
  on-line data collection/
   recording, 80
  pass/fail criteria, 82
  reinforcement for fluency, 83
  types of reinforcers, 83, 84
  use of punishment, 76, 79, 82,
   94, 96
 establishing fluent speech, 35, 81,
  143
 function of reinforcement, 35, 143
 gentle onset of voice, 86
 graduated length of utterance, 40,
  57
 modifying attitudes, 54, 57-58, 64,
  88
 rate control, 58, 84-86
 reducing physical concomitants, 55
 reducing word avoidance, 55
 sentence formulation, 52
 simplifying speaking activities, 35,
  37, 87
 syllable and motor support
  training, 51, 66-67
 transfer group, 97
Time out studies, 77
Trigger conditions in stuttering, 14,
 16-17, 19
Twinning in stutterers, 4, 8

Uncertainty/doubt about speaking:
 as targets of intervention, 28, 35,
  37
 role in disfluency and stuttering,
  22, 23, 24, 25
 sources of, 27, 28